300 SINGLE BEST ANSWER
QUESTIONS FOR
MEDICAL AND
SURGICAL FINALS

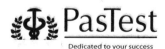
PasTest
Dedicated to your success

In Memory Of

Kasturben Ramniklal Gohil

Ashok Ramniklal Gohil

&

Jamuben Mulji Bhundia

Hemraj Mulji Bhundia

300 SINGLE BEST ANSWER QUESTIONS FOR MEDICAL AND SURGICAL FINALS
SECOND EDITION

Dr Satyen Gohil BSc MBBS
Core Medical Trainee
Kent Oncology Centre
Maidstone Hospital
Kent

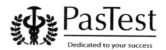

PasTest
Dedicated to your success

© 2009 PASTEST LTD
Egerton Court
Parkgate Estate
Knutsford
Cheshire
WA16 8DX
Telephone: 01565 752000

First published 2007, Second edition 2009

ISBN: 1905635540

ISBN: 9781905635542

A catalogue record for this book is available from the British Library.

PasTest Revision Books and Intensive Courses

PasTest has been established in the field of undergraduate and postgraduate medical education since 1972, providing revision books and intensive study courses for doctors preparing for their professional examinations.

Books and courses are available for:

Medical undergraduates, MRCGP, MRCP Parts 1 and 2, MRCPCH Parts 1 and 2, MRCS, MRCOG Parts 1 and 2, DRCOG, DCH, FRCA, Dentistry.

For further details contact:

PasTest, Freepost, Knutsford, Cheshire WA16 7BR

Tel: 01565 752000   Fax: 01565 650264

www.pastest.co.uk   enquires@pastest.co.uk

Text prepared by Carnegie Book Production, Lancaster, UK

Printed and bound in the UK by Athenaeum Press, Gateshead

CONTENTS

He who asks a question may look momentarily stupid ...

.... but he who does not will remain forever ignorant

Chinese Proverb

ACKNOWLEDGEMENT

To Diya, for everything ...

PREFACE TO THE SECOND EDITION

Revising for medical exams can be extremely daunting, with endless hours of revision and practice questions never seeming to prepare me or my friends for the sorts of questions which were actually encountered when we took the exam. With that in mind I sought to create a book which aimed to reflect the complexity of the questions that are devised by examiners while encouraging those using the book to read around the subject and gain a wider knowledge base and understanding of medicine in general.

The second edition draws on the strengths of the first and is revised to take into account comments and feedback from colleagues, friends and, most importantly, those who have used the first edition of the book, taken their finals and passed, to create a better and more relevant guide for exam preparation.

I can't promise that this book has all of the questions that will be encountered in your final exams but hope that it does help you prepare for them, impart some knowledge along the way, and, most importantly, makes you feel more confident when you turn over the first page of the exam paper.

Good luck!

Satyen Gohil

London, 2009

FOREWORD TO THE FIRST EDITION

Dr Satyen Gohil qualified in medicine from the King's College London School of Medicine in July 2006. He excelled as an undergraduate, obtaining a first class BSc and distinctions in the Final MB BS examinations, and has been appointed to one of our highly competitive academic foundation year 1 posts in King's College Hospital NHS Foundation Trust. In this role, it has been a pleasure to observe his academic excellence providing the basis for the development of clinical and communication skills, which will ensure that he excels as a medical practitioner in the future.

As a newly qualified doctor and with his academic track record, he is eminently well qualified to evaluate the educational material needs of those preparing for the final MB BS examination and to seek to address these as he now does in this book. Clinical medicine is a fast-moving and rapidly developing field and the knowledge base continues to grow accordingly. Trying to grasp the key elements and understand them and ensuring that one does not become mesmerised by irrelevant minutiae is critical. In addition, recognising that a significant part of the successful preparation process for the examination is understanding the style and processes of the examination and becoming competent at them is also critical to achieving success at this final hurdle. With these characteristics in mind Dr Gohil has sought to develop a book of questions for final-year medical students which uses scenario-based and knowledge-based questions in the style now commonly used across medical schools in the UK. The questions are appropriate to the final examination and will certainly challenge students' knowledge and encourage them to both think and go searching for information. The answers given in the book are well written and helpful and the explanations certainly provide appropriate and sufficient information.

This is a timely book, which fills a gap in the revision process for students preparing for the Final MB BS examination and will undoubtedly be useful and helpful to them. Dr Gohil has identified a real need in the educational material for medical students at this stage of their studies and he is to be commended for his efforts.

Alan M. McGregor

Professor of Medicine
Campus Dean – Denmark Hill
King's College School of Medicine

ABBREVIATIONS

AF	atrial fibrillation
αFP	alpha-fetoprotein
ABG	arterial blood gas
ACE	angiotensin-converting enzyme
ACTH	adrenocorticotrophic hormone
ADH	antidiuretic hormone
AFB	acid-fast bacilli
AIDS	acquired immunodeficiency syndrome
ALP	alkaline phosphatase
ALT	alanine aminotransferase
AMT	abbreviated mental test
ANA	antinuclear antibody
ANCA	anti-neutrophil cytoplasmic antibody
APACHE	acute physiology and chronic health evaluation
AST	aspartate aminotransferase
BCG	bacille Calmette-Guerin
BHL	bilateral hilar lymphadenopathy
BMI	body mass index
BNP	B-type natriuretic peptide
CEA	carcinoembryonic antigen
CDT	*Clostridium difficile* toxin
CIN	cervical intraepithelial neoplasia
CLL	chronic lymphocytic leukaemia
COMT	catechol-O-methyltransferase
COPD	chronic obstructive pulmonary disease
CPAP	continuous positive airway pressure (ventilation)
CPR	cardiopulmonary resuscitation
CRP	C-reactive protein
CSF	cerebrospinal fluid
dsDNA	double-stranded DNA
DVT	deep vein thrombosis

ERCP	endoscopic retrograde cholangiopancreatography
ESR	erythrocyte sedimentation rate
F1	Foundation year 1 doctor
F2	Foundation year 2 doctor
FEV1	forced expiratory volume in 1 second
FFP	fresh frozen plasma
FH	familial hypercholesterolaemia
FiO$_2$	fraction of inspired oxygen
FVC	forced vital capacity
G6PD	glucose-6-phosphate dehydrogenase
GCS	Glasgow coma scale
GFR	glomerular filtration rate
GORD	gastro-oesophageal reflux disease
GTN	glyceryl trinitrate
HAART	highly active antiretroviral treatment
hCG	human chorionic gonadotrophin
HDL	high-density lipoprotein
HDU	High-Dependency Unit
HLA	human leukocyte antigen
HONKC	hyper-osmolar non-ketotic coma
HSP	Henoch–Schönlein purpura
HUS	haemolytic uraemic syndrome
IV	intravenous
IVDU	intravenous drug user
J	joules
JVP	jugular venous pressure
LBBB	left bundle branch block
LDH	lactate dehydrogenase
LDL	low-density lipoprotein
LFT	liver function test
LTOT	long-term oxygen therapy
MCV	mean cell volume
MHC	major histocompatibility complex
MMSE	mini mental state examination
MRI	magnetic resonance imaging
MRSA	methicillin-resistant *Staphylococcus aureus*
MSH	melanocyte-stimulating hormone
NAC	N-acetylcysteine
NG	nasogastric

NICE	formerly: National Institute for Clinical Excellence currently: National Institute for Health and Clinical Excellence
NMDA	N-methyl-D-aspartate
NSAIDs	non-steroidal anti-inflammatory drugs
NSTEMI	non-ST-elevation myocardial infarction
$PaCO_2$	partial pressure of carbon dioxide
PaO_2	partial pressure of oxygen
PCA	patient-controlled analgesia
PCI	primary coronary intervention
PCP	*Pneumocystis carinii* pneumonia
PCR	polymerase chain reaction
p.r.n.	*pro re nata*
PSA	prostate-specific antigen
PSC	primary sclerosing cholangitis
PSGN	post-streptococcal glomerulonephritis
RAS	renal artery stenosis
RBBB	right bundle branch block
SIADH	syndrome of inappropriate ADH secretion
SLE	systemic lupus erythematosus
STEMI	ST-elevation myocardial infarction
STD	sexually transmitted disease
TFTs	thyroid function tests
U	units
UC	ulcerative colitis
V/Q	ventilation/perfusion
WCC	white cell count

QUESTIONS

SECTION 1:
SCENARIO-BASED QUESTIONS

Scenario 1

A 62-year-old patient presents to the Emergency Department with worsening leg swelling that has developed over the previous few months. She reports that her GP has tried to help with water tablets but that they have not helped and have caused incontinence instead. Over this time she has found herself becoming easily tired and requiring increasing help from her daughters. Her past medical history is significant for hypertension and a previous non-ST-segment-elevation myocardial infarction (NSTEMI) a year ago. She had an echocardiogram performed 2 months ago which showed normal right and left ventricular size and function, with an estimated ejection fraction of 50%–60%. There was some wall motion abnormality of the inferior wall but this was not thought to be significant. Her medications include aspirin, furosemide, amlodipine and ramipril.

On examination the patient has obvious facial puffiness, bilateral swollen legs with pitting oedema to the shins and an element of sacral oedema. Her legs are erythematous with some weeping and are slightly tender. Blood tests show:

Sodium	140 mmol/l
Potassium	5.2 mmol/l
Creatinine	174 µmol/l ↑
Urea	7.8 mmol/l –
Corrected calcium	2.21 mmol/l –
Albumin	18 g/l ↓
Cholesterol	6.1 mmol/l ↑

Haemoglobin	12.8 g/dl
White cell count	10.2×10^9/l
Neutrophils	7.3×10^9/l
Platelets	122×10^9/l
INR	1.1
Urine dipstick:	
Leukocytes	+
Nitrites	Negative
Protein	+ + +
Ketones	+
Blood	+

S1.1 Which ONE of the following would be most appropriate, given this information?

○ A Repeat echocardiogram
○ B Thyroid function tests
○ C Doppler ultrasound of the lower limbs
○ D Antibiotics
○ E Urine analysis

S1.2 Which ONE of the following is true with regard to the underlying diagnosis in this patient?

○ A Heparin is absolutely contraindicated
○ B The ACE inhibitor should be stopped immediately
○ C There is increased susceptibility to infections
○ D Hypercholesterolaemia is not linked to the underlying diagnosis
○ E Fluid and salt should be restricted but protein intake should be greatly increased

ANSWERS ON PAGE 161

Scenario 2

You are the F1 doctor on the Medical Assessment Unit and are reviewing a father and his two children who present with worsening headaches, myalgia and lethargy. The two children have also complained of stomach aches. This problem has been present for the past week and has been getting gradually worse. The children's mother, who also suffers from headaches, has been visiting a distant aunt over the last week and has been feeling better away from home.

There is no past medical history of note but the father is unsure of whether the children have had all their childhood immunisations. On examination the father is comfortable at rest, with a pulse of 90 bpm, blood pressure 115/78 mmHg, a respiratory rate of 25 per minute, oxygen saturations of 100% on room air and a clear chest, with no cardiac murmurs.

S2.1 Which ONE of the following is the most likely diagnosis?

O   A   Unintentional poisoning
O   B   Influenza
O   C   Non-specific viral infection
O   D   Family difficulties
O   E   Encephalitis

S2.2 Which ONE of the following is the most appropriate?

O   A   Viral swabs and serology
O   B   Referral to the on-call social services team
O   C   Reassure and discharge
O   D   Chest X-ray
O   E   Commence oxygen therapy

ANSWERS ON PAGE 162

5

Scenario 3

You are the admitting doctor on the acute medical team and are referred a patient by the GP with a creatinine of 547 μmol/l, which has risen from a baseline of 85 μmol/l 2 months previously. The patient describes feeling generally unwell with whole-body myalgia and arthralgia. On examination he has a soft ejection systolic murmur over the aortic area, bibasal crepitations on auscultation, and a soft and non-tender abdomen with no suprapubic bladder palpable. Urine is concentrated and dark, with dipstick showing the presence of protein + and blood + + +.

The patient has a past history of ischaemic heart disease which has required three coronary artery stents following a myocardial infarction 2 years previously. He has recently been found to be in atrial fibrillation, for which he taking amiodarone 200 mg once daily, in addition to his aspirin 75 mg once daily, ramipril 5 mg once daily, isosorbide mononitrate modified release 120 mg once daily, furosemide 40 mg once daily and simvastatin 40 mg at night.

S3.1: Which ONE of the following is the most appropriate?

- A Echocardiogram
- B Renal ultrasound
- C Prednisolone
- D Renal biopsy
- E Intravenous fluids

S3.2: Which ONE of the following is the underlying cause?

- A Interstitial nephritis
- B Volume depletion
- C Drug interaction
- D Obstructive nephropathy
- E Congestive cardiac failure

ANSWERS ON PAGE 163

Scenario 4

A 65-year-old patient presents to you in general practice with a painful right lower leg. On questioning, he tells you that the pain has been present for a few months but he has not sought any medical advice for it. His past medical history is significant only for type 2 diabetes, for which he is on insulin. On examination he appears systemically well. Examination of the right lower limb shows a curvature of the tibia with overlying erythema, and palpation reveals it to be much warmer than the left leg.

S4.1: Which ONE of the following conditions is the patient suffering from?

○ A Osteomyelitis
○ B Paget's disease
○ C Sarcoma
○ D Skeletal metastasis
○ E Charcot's joint

S4.2: Which ONE of the following is the most appropriate in this patient?

○ A Intravenous antibiotics
○ B Bone biopsy with or without excision
○ C Immobilisation
○ D CT chest, abdomen and pelvis
○ E Osteoclast inhibition

Scenario 5

A 76-year-old woman presents with a 2-week history of nausea and vomiting, resulting in some loss of weight and 'just not feeling herself'. She also describes feeling generally weak, easily fatigued and seeing a yellow hue around lights. She has a past history of atrial fibrillation, hypertension and congestive cardiac failure. Her full blood count shows a haemoglobin of 10.4 g/dl, an MCV of 99.2 fl, and a normal white cell count and differential. Her creatinine has come back as 261 μmol/l from a baseline of 150 μmol/l a few weeks previously, with a sodium of 133 mmol/l and a potassium of 4.2 mmol/l.

S5.1: Which ONE of the following medications is most likely to have led to the above presentation?

○ A Amiodarone
○ B Diltiazem
○ C Digoxin
○ D Flecainide
○ E Furosemide

S5.2: Out of the following investigations, which ONE is the most appropriate in patients with the above diagnosis?

○ A Sodium level
○ B Albumin:creatinine ratio
○ C Potassium levels
○ D Calcium levels
○ E 24-hour tape

ANSWERS ON PAGE 165

Scenario 6

You are attending a genetic counselling session at the regional Genetics Unit.

S6.1: A patient with sickle cell disease is considering having a child with her partner, who has sickle cell trait. What is the probability that the child will have sickle cell disease?

- ○ A 25%
- ○ B 33%
- ○ C 50%
- ○ D 75%
- ○ E 100%

S6.2: Mrs Smith is the sister of a patient who suffers from disease X, which is inherited in an autosomal recessive manner and which has a carrier frequency of 1 in 10 in the general population. The carriers of disease X are not adversely affected and are phenotypically identical to the normal population. Mrs Smith is fit and well and is thinking about having children with her husband, who is not affected by disease X and who has no family history of disease X. Mrs Smith wants to know what the probability of her child suffering from disease X is. Which ONE of the following is the correct answer?

- ○ A 0
- ○ B 1/15
- ○ C 1/20
- ○ D 1/60
- ○ E 1/80

S6.3 **You are reviewing a family with a history of Huntingdon's disease. Which of the following statements is true?**

○ A Autosomal dominant condition on chromosome 5

○ B Due to repeat of the CAC trinucleotide

○ C Has full penetrance in offspring

○ D Tetrabenazine prevents progression of the disease

○ E Encapatone has been shown to be beneficial

ANSWER ON PAGE 167

Scenario 7

A 64-year-old retired estate agent is brought into the Emergency Department in a confused and agitated state. His wife states that over the last month he has lost a considerable amount of weight and has complained of increasing fatigue. He also has been passing water far more frequently recently and has started to take a jug of water to bed at night.

His routine blood tests are returned as:

Sodium	150 mmol/l
Potassium	5 mmol/l
Creatinine	105 µmol/l
Urea	9 mmol/l
Calcium	2.5 mmol/l
Albumin	45 g/l
Glucose	27 mmol/l
Chloride	90 mmol/l
CRP	5 mg/l

S7.1 What is the calculated plasma osmolality in mosmol/kg?

- A 190
- B 254
- C 337
- D 346
- E 414

S7.2 **Which of the following is the single most important treatment in this patient?**

○ A 10 units of fast-acting insulin stat

○ B Insulin sliding scale

○ C Intramuscular glucagon

○ D Colloid fluid resuscitation

○ E Saline fluid administration

S7.3 **In the diagnosis of the *underlying condition* which has led to the above presentation, which ONE of the following statements is true?**

○ A In the above patient an oral glucose tolerance test is essential to establish the underlying diagnosis

○ B In the above patient two separate fasting blood glucose levels greater than or equal to 7.0 mmol/l are needed to establish the underlying diagnosis

○ C In any patient a single random blood glucose of 11.0 mmol/l is sufficient to establish the diagnosis

○ D In any patient a blood glucose of 7.9 mmol/l 2 hours following an oral glucose tolerance test implies impaired glucose tolerance

○ E Measurement of HbA1c is routinely used to establish the diagnosis

Scenario 8

A 55-year-old schoolteacher with known breast cancer presents with increasing confusion, non-localising abdominal pain, fatigue and a history of increasing thirst and weight loss. She also complains of pain in the small of the back and tenderness on the right side of her chest.

S8.1 Which of the following treatments is *least* indicated in the management of this condition?

- ○ A Fluid rehydration
- ○ B Furosemide
- ○ C Pamidronate infusion
- ○ D Bendroflumethiazide
- ○ E Calcitonin

S8.2 How would this clinical condition manifest itself initially on an ECG?

- ○ A Shortened QT interval
- ○ B Presence of J waves
- ○ C Presence of U waves
- ○ D Widening of the QRS complex
- ○ E Prolonged QT interval

questions

S8.3   Which ONE of the following is true with regard to breast cancer?

○   A   The National Breast Screening Programme in the UK invites all women registered at a general practice for screening between the ages of 45 and 70

○   B   Approximately 1500 lives are saved annually by the NHS breast screening programme in the UK

○   C   Triple assessment of history and examination, mammography and histology/cytology is used in all patients with suspected breast cancer

○   D   *HER2* is a tumour suppressor gene that is targeted by trastuzumab

○   E   Tamoxifen is a selective oestrogen receptor agonist

ANSWERS ON PAGES 170–171

Scenario 9

A 70-year-old lady is brought into the Emergency Department by her worried neighbours, who report her not being her usual self. On examination she looks unwell, is confused and complains of a headache. She is pyrexial, does not tolerate examination of pupillary reflexes and flexion of the neck causes hip flexion.

S9.1 What is the most likely organism involved?

○ A Gram-negative intracellular diplococci
○ B Acid-fast-bacilli (AFB)
○ C Alpha-haemolytic streptococci
○ D Coagulase-positive staphylococci
○ E Gram-negative bacilli

S9.2 What is the most appropriate antibiotic for this patient from the list below?

○ A Benzylpenicillin
○ B Rifampicin
○ C Metronidazole
○ D Ciprofloxacin
○ E Ceftriaxone

Another patient with a similar complaint is brought into the Emergency Department and after taking a history, examination and performing appropriate investigations you suspect cryptococcal meningitis.

S9.3 **Which ONE of the following investigations would be most appropriate in a patient with suspected cryptococcal meningitis?**

○ A CSF virology

○ B India ink staining of CSF

○ C Silver staining of CSF

○ D Microscopy of CSF

○ E AFB staining of CSF

S9.4 **In a patient with confirmed *Cryptococcus* meningitis what is the most important investigation to perform prior to initiating standard treatment?**

○ A Liver function tests

○ B Renal function tests

○ C Full blood count and differentials

○ D CT head

○ E ECG

ANSWERS ON PAGE 172

Scenario 10

A patient presents to her general practice with a history of joint pains, tiredness, oral ulcers and a rash on her hands and the front of her chest. Her husband, who accompanied her to the consultation, states how he has noticed her face to be brighter and redder than usual. Of note she was recently started on anti-tuberculosis treatment.

S10.1 Which ONE of the following is most likely to have caused the above symptoms in this patient?

- ○ A Isoniazid
- ○ B Rifampicin
- ○ C Pyridoxine
- ○ D Ethambutol
- ○ E Pyrazinamide

S10.2 Which ONE of the following antibodies is present in 90% of patients with the above condition?

- ○ A Anti-nuclear antibody
- ○ B Anti-double-stranded DNA antibody
- ○ C Anti-mitochondrial antibody
- ○ D Classical anti-neutrophil cytoplasmic antibody
- ○ E Anti-histone antibody

S10.3 Which ONE of the following tests is *least* useful in monitoring the activity of the idiopathic form of the disease?

- ○ A Erythrocyte sedimentation rate
- ○ B Complement levels
- ○ C C-reactive protein
- ○ D Blood pressure measurement
- ○ E Urinalysis

ANSWERS ON PAGE 173

17

Scenario 11

A 30-year-old fitness instructor comes to the General Medical Clinic with a 3-month history of malaise, lethargy and weight loss. On further questioning he reports intermittent colicky abdominal pain with diarrhoea, mucus and blood per rectum. On examination he is a tall thin man; cardiovascular, respiratory and abdominal examination are unremarkable and rectal examination reveals a few anal skin tags. Examination of the mouth reveals some aphthous ulcers.

S11.1 Which ONE of the following treatment options is *least* effective in the acute management of active disease in patients with the above condition?

○ A Intravenous fluids

○ B Hydrocortisone

○ C Metronidazole

○ D Azathioprine

○ E Elemental diet

S11.2 Which ONE of the following findings would not occur in patients with the above disease?

○ A Rose-thorn ulceration on sigmoidoscopy

○ B Transmural granulomatous inflammation

○ C Colovesical fistula formation

○ D Toxic dilatation

○ E Osteomalacia

ANSWERS ON PAGE 174

S11.3 **In patients with inflammatory bowel disease which ONE of the following extra-gastrointestinal conditions is more commonly associated with ulcerative colitis than with Crohn's disease?**

○ A Gallstones
○ B Renal stones
○ C Uveitis
○ D Venous thrombosis
○ E Erythema nodosum

Scenario 12

A 17-year-old student is brought in by ambulance complaining of shortness of breath. He is known to be asthmatic and takes salbutamol and beclometasone regularly. This is his first hospital admission with an acute asthma attack.

S12.1 Which ONE of the following features suggests a diagnosis *other than* severe asthma?

- A   Pulse of 115/minute
- B   Inability to complete sentences
- C   Respiratory rate of 27/minute
- D   Inability to perform peak flow measurement
- E   Blood pressure of 90/60 mmHg

S12.2 After ensuring stability of his airway, breathing and circulation, what is the most appropriate first-line treatment in this patient?

- A   Controlled oxygen therapy with an FiO_2 of 24%
- B   Salbutamol 500 micrograms nebulised
- C   Terbutaline 10 mg nebulised
- D   Hydrocortisone 200 mg intravenously
- E   Continuous positive airway pressure ventilation

S12.3 Which ONE of the following statements is *not* true?

O   A   Asthma affects over 5 million children in the UK

O   B   Gastro-oesophageal reflux disease is associated with asthma

O   C   Asthma may be the presenting feature of an underlying vasculitis

O   D   During childhood more males are affected than females, with this ratio reversing in adults aged 40 to 50

O   E   During an asthma attack, while waiting for an ambulance, it is advisable to keep taking salbutamol every minute for 5 minutes or until a response is obtained

S12.4 Prior to this admission he was taking one of his medications far more frequently than usual and noticed that he had developed a tremor of his hands. Which ONE of these statements is true with regard to this medication?

O   A   At high doses he should be advised to rinse his mouth out after use

O   B   The medication is known to cause hypokalaemia

O   C   Drug levels are useful to assess drug compliance

O   D   The medication is known as Atrovent

O   E   Ipratropium is as useful as this medication in the chronic treatment of asthma

Scenario 13

A 56-year-old businessman returns from a trip to Thailand complaining of pain on passing water accompanied by a profuse discharge 'down below'. He denies any other symptoms.

S13.1 Which ONE of the following is most likely to be the causative agent?

○ A *Neisseria gonorrhoeae*

○ B *Chlamydia trachomatis*

○ C *Trichomonas vaginalis*

○ D *Treponema pallidum*

○ E *Candida albicans*

S13.2 Which ONE of the following appearances would be most likely to be seen in the above patient on microscopy?

○ A Intracellular Gram-negative rods

○ B Comma-shaped organisms on silver staining

○ C Organism not detectable on microscopy

○ D Motile parasites

○ E Gram-negative diplococci

S13.3 The patient is successfully treated but returns 2 weeks later complaining of the same symptoms. Which ONE of the following is the most likely diagnosis?

○ A Co-existent infection

○ B Bacterial resistance against antibiotics

○ C Incomplete eradication of the pathogen

○ D Re-acquisition of the same pathogen

○ E None of the above

ANSWERS ON PAGE 177

S13.4 A different patient presents to the Sexually Transmitted Disease Clinic with a history of tender inguinal lymph nodes. On further questioning he describes pain around the anus, bloody diarrhoea, tenesmus and purulent discharge. The patient is a homosexual who says he rarely uses a condom. On examination there are multiple fluctuant inguinal lymph nodes palpable, which are beginning to coalesce, with a few beginning to break down and discharge. Which ONE of the following is the most likely diagnosis?

○ A *Treponema pallidum*

○ B *Klebsiella granulomatis*

○ C *Haemophilus ducreyi*

○ D *Chlamydia trachomatis*

○ E Underlying inflammatory bowel disease

Scenario 14

A 68-year-old retired head-teacher comes to your general practice surgery complaining of back pain which is quite similar to an episode she had last year. Two years ago she had fractured her ulna and radius after a simple fall. On examination she has a marked kyphosis and is tender over the mid-thoracic spine. Inflammatory and neoplastic lesions have been excluded.

S14.1 Which ONE of the following does *not* increase the risk of developing the underlying condition which has led to the above?

○ A Multiple myeloma

○ B Myxoedema

○ C Hyperparathyroidism

○ D Hypogonadism

○ E Anorexia nervosa

S14.2 Which ONE of the following statements is true with regard to the underlying diagnosis?

○ A Routine blood tests for calcium, phosphate and alkaline phosphatase are usually returned as abnormal in the above condition

○ B Peak bone mass is attained between the second and third decades of life

○ C A T-score of between 1 and 2.5 represents osteopenia

○ D An obstructive pattern on spirometry would be expected in patients with advanced-stage disease

○ E The gold standard for diagnosing the above condition is an isotope bone scan

S14.3 Which ONE of the following statements is true?

○ A Parathyroid hormone increases the levels of circulating calcium and phosphate in the body

○ B The most active metabolite of vitamin D is produced by the liver

○ C The average diet should include 100 mg of calcium and 100 IU of vitamin D per day

○ D Osteoporosis is implicated in over 150 000 fractures annually in the UK

○ E Secondary osteoporosis is more common than primary osteoporosis

ANSWER ON PAGE 179

Scenario 15

A 28-year-old patient presents with an erythematous rash which shows concentric rings like target lesions. The rash is predominantly on the palms and soles, with blistering present.

S15.1 Which ONE of the following is the most likely in the above patient?

- ○ A Pyoderma gangrenosum
- ○ B Erythema nodosum
- ○ C Erythema marginatum
- ○ D Erythema multiforme
- ○ E Erythema chronicum migrans

S15.2 Which ONE of the following is the commonest identifiable cause of the above rash?

- ○ A Carcinoma
- ○ B Herpes zoster
- ○ C Herpes simplex
- ○ D *Mycoplasma pneumoniae*
- ○ E Sulphonamides

ANSWERS ON PAGE 180

Scenario 16

You are working as a junior doctor in general practice and are reviewing a range of patients with hypertension.

S16.1 A patient with persistently raised blood pressure despite adequate lifestyle modifications was started on a new medication. When you review her in clinic she describes how her family have noticed her smile to have changed. On examination she has obvious gum hypertrophy. Which ONE medication from the following list is most likely to cause the above side-effect?

- A Phenytoin
- B Ramipril
- C Bumetanide
- D Indapamide
- E Nifedipine

S16.2 A patient with persistently raised blood pressure despite adequate lifestyle modification was started on a new medication. When you review him in clinic he seems hesitant and nervous. He has been on treatment for a number of months but his medication does not seem to have had any effect on controlling his blood pressure. He states that his hands and feet are colder than in the past and on direct questioning admits that he has difficulty performing in the bedroom with his partner. Which ONE of the following is most likely?

- A Non-compliance
- B Non-concordance
- C Attention-seeking behaviour
- D Underlying diabetes mellitus
- E None of the above

S16.3 A patient with persistently raised blood pressure despite adequate lifestyle modifications has been tried on a number of medications, all of which have had disappointing results on his blood pressure management. Two weeks after starting a new medication his blood tests showed a substantial decrease in the value obtained using the Cockcroft–Gault formula. However, this recovered satisfactorily when treatment was discontinued. Which ONE of the following would you initially request to delineate the underlying abnormality?

- A Renal biopsy
- B MRI imaging
- C CT imaging
- D Ultrasound
- E Angiography

S16.4 In the above patient which ONE of the following is considered to be the gold-standard diagnostic test?

- A Renal biopsy
- B MRI imaging
- C CT imaging
- D Ultrasound
- E Angiography

ANSWERS ON PAGE 182

S16.5 **A patient with diagnosed type 2 diabetes is started on medication for his high blood pressure, which remains stubbornly high. He is started on appropriate treatment, but notices that his smoker's cough, which he has had for a number of years, is getting progressively worse. Despite your best efforts on repeated occasions he refuses to give up smoking. What is the most appropriate treatment in this patient?**

○ A Losartan
○ B Nicotine replacement
○ C Atenolol
○ D Amlodipine
○ E Enalapril

questions

Scenario 17

You are working as an F1 in general practice and a slim patient with tiredness, diarrhoea and a rash comes to see you. He has been to the Dermatology Clinic and a report from the clinic has been faxed to you from the local hospital.

It states that there was patchy granular IgA deposition along the basement membrane and IgA located at the tips of the dermal papillae on direct immunofluorescence.

The diagnosis section on the fax has not transmitted well and you cannot make out what is written.

S17.1 What is the most likely diagnosis in the above patient?

- A Pemphigus vulgaris
- B Bullous pemphigoid
- C Epidermolysis bullosa
- D Dermatomyositis
- E Dermatitis herpetiformis

S17.2 What is the most suitable treatment option in the above patient?

- A Non-drug treatment
- B Dapsone
- C Sulfapyridine
- D Azathioprine
- E Prednisolone

ANSWERS ON PAGE 183

S17.3 **A different patient is started on a medication that is used in the treatment of the above condition. She develops marked jaundice associated with dark urine and states that she feels weak and tired. On examination she has obvious jaundice, is feverish and has a tachycardia. Which ONE of the following conditions would best account for the above presentation?**

○   A   Sickle cell disease

○   B   Thalassaemia

○   C   Hereditary spherocytosis

○   D   Glucose-6-phosphate dehydrogenase (G6PD) deficiency

○   E   Concurrent malaria infection

questions

Scenario 18

A 59-year-old airline pilot was admitted for osteomyelitis and prompt intravenous antibiotic therapy was instituted. He remained in hospital for a further 2 weeks but developed copious offensive diarrhoea, which required intravenous fluid replacement.

S18.1 What is the most useful test in establishing the diagnosis in the above patient?

○ A Stool culture and sensitivity
○ B Stool toxin analysis
○ C Stool microscopy
○ D Stool PCR
○ E Sigmoidoscopy

S18.2 Which ONE of the following best describes the organism involved?

○ A Gram-positive rod
○ B Gram-negative rod
○ C Parasite
○ D Gram-positive coccus
○ E Gram-negative coccus

S18.3 Which ONE of the following is most suitable in the first-line treatment of the above patient?

○ A Vancomycin
○ B Ciprofloxacin
○ C Gentamicin
○ D Metronidazole
○ E Penicillin V

questions

Scenario 19

A 23-year-old student comes into hospital as part of the regular treatment for his condition. He was first brought to see you at a young age after his GP noticed he was not gaining weight adequately. In addition he was noted to be an ill child and was always developing colds. The mother distinctly remembers that he had difficulty passing his first motions after he was born.

S19.1 What is the approximate carrier frequency of the above disease?

O   A   1/5
O   B   1/25
O   C   1/200
O   D   1/500
O   E   1/2500

S19.2 At the age of 18 years he presented with severe pneumonia productive of green sputum, which indicated the acquisition of a pathogen the doctors had been worried about for a number of years. What is the most likely pathogen?

O   A   *Staphylococcus aureus*
O   B   *Klebsiella pneumoniae*
O   C   *Pseudomonas aeruginosa*
O   D   *Streptococcus pneumoniae*
O   E   *Mycoplasma pneumoniae*

S19.3 Which ONE of the following antibiotics is most suitable for the above patient with the above pathogen?

○   A   Ciprofloxacin

○   B   Benzylpenicillin

○   C   Cefuroxime

○   D   Erythromycin

○   E   Tetracycline

Scenario 20

You are undertaking a special study module in the Department of Epidemiology. During this time you analyse the relationship between breast cancer and use of substance X. You compare data of 500 women with breast cancer and 500 women without breast cancer and investigate their previous history to analyse their use of substance X.

S20.1 Which ONE of the following best describes this study?

○   A   Case–control study

○   B   Blinded randomised controlled trial

○   C   Non-blinded randomised controlled trial

○   D   Longitudinal analysis

○   E   Cohort study

While investigating another scenario you notice that the data are normally distributed.

S20.2 How many standard deviations from the mean would include 95% of the population?

○   A   0.5

○   B   3

○   C   1

○   D   1.5

○   E   2

On elective in America you take part in a research programme investigating the usefulness of a new blood test in the diagnosis of heart failure. You compare this test with the gold standard. You recruited 500 people into the study, 300 of whom tested positive on the blood test but only 250 of whom had proved heart failure; 150 were negative both on blood testing and the gold standard; 50 people tested negative on the blood test but actually did have heart failure.

S20.3 Which ONE of the following is most likely to be considered the gold-standard investigation for heart failure?

- ○ A ECG
- ○ B BNP measurement
- ○ C Echocardiography
- ○ D Angiography
- ○ E Exercise testing

S20.4 What is the sensitivity of the blood test?

- ○ A 83%
- ○ B 72%
- ○ C 91%
- ○ D 33%
- ○ E 15%

ANSWERS ON PAGES 186–187

Scenario 21

You are the F1 on call over the weekend and get bleeped at 10pm to be told that one of the patients in the general medicine wards is going into 'acute renal failure'.

S21.1 Which ONE of the following is *least* useful in the *initial* assessment of the above patient?

○ A   JVP
○ B   Ultrasound
○ C   Serum urea and creatinine
○ D   ABG
○ E   Urine output

You are asked to see another patient with acute renal failure.

S21.2 On examination you note the patient does not seem to be himself and has a thready and irregular pulse. You arrange for an urgent ECG, which shows tented T waves and widening of the QRS complex. What is the most appropriate measure to correct the underlying abnormality?

○ A   Dialysis
○ B   10 ml of 10% calcium gluconate over 10 minutes
○ C   Calcium resonium
○ D   50% dextrose with 10 units Actrapid insulin
○ E   50 ml 8.4% bicarbonate via a central line

Scenario 22

You are the on-call F1 doctor and are bleeped because a patient has collapsed in the Outpatient Department. You are the first to reach him and assess his airway, breathing and circulation. His airway is patent but there is no evidence of breathing or circulation. You start CPR and wait for the arrival of the resuscitation team.

S22.1 What is the correct relationship between compressions and breaths?

- ○ A 15 compressions to 1 breath
- ○ B 15 compressions to 2 breaths
- ○ C 30 compressions to 1 breath
- ○ D 30 compressions to 2 breaths
- ○ E 10 compressions to 1 breath

S22.2 The resuscitation team arrive and you attach the electrodes to the patient, which reveals ventricular fibrillation. What is the next step?

- ○ A Defibrillate at 200 J
- ○ B Continue CPR for 1 minute
- ○ C Give patient 1 mg adrenaline (epinephrine)
- ○ D Defibrillate at 360 J
- ○ E Give atropine

S22.3 The shock you give does not convert the rhythm to sinus rhythm. What is the next step?

- ○ A Charge defibrillator at 300 J
- ○ B Charge defibrillator at 360 J
- ○ C Charge defibrillator at 400 J
- ○ D Resume CPR for 2 minutes
- ○ E Resume CPR for 1 minute

ANSWERS ON PAGE 189

S22.4 After a couple of cycles of CPR the rhythm changes to sinus rhythm but the rate is 30 with a blood pressure of 75/40 mmHg. What is the next appropriate step?

O   A   Adrenaline

O   B   Atropine

O   C   Glucagon

O   D   Verapamil

O   E   Lidocaine

S22.5 The above step fails to raise the heart rate or the blood pressure and the patient starts deteriorating rapidly. What should be done immediately?

O   A   Transvenous pacing

O   B   Transcutaneous pacing

O   C   Synchronised DC cardioversion at 100 J

O   D   Synchronised DC cardioversion at 200 J

O   E   Intra-aortic balloon counterpulsation

ANSWERS ON PAGE 189

Scenario 23

A 20-year-old student is brought into the Emergency Department after being found with an empty bottle of paracetamol tablets next to her. Her mother states that she recently broke up with her long-term boyfriend and that this overdose is not in keeping with her usual character.

S23.1 Which ONE of the following statements is true?

○ A Paracetamol poisoning is the second most commonly encountered drug overdose in the UK

○ B The hepatotoxic dose of paracetamol is taken as 150 mg/kg for high-risk patients

○ C Paracetamol overdose leads to approximately 2000 deaths per year

○ D Activated charcoal is better than gastric lavage in the above situation

○ E N-acetylcysteine is approximately 75% useful in preventing significant hepatic impairment if given within 12 hours of ingestion

S23.2 Which ONE of the following statements is true?

○ A High-risk patients are those in whom hepatic glutathione reserves are increased

○ B Patients with anorexia nervosa should be treated using the low-risk treatment line

○ C 1% of patients develop an allergic reaction to N-acetylcysteine

○ D Methionine is an alternative to N-acetylcysteine

○ E Serum albumin is the best indicator for severity of liver damage

ANSWERS ON PAGES 190–191

S23.3 The factors below all increase the risk of hepatotoxicity secondary to paracetamol overdose EXCEPT?

○ A Phenytoin
○ B Cystic fibrosis
○ C Human immunodeficiency virus
○ D Cimetidine
○ E Long-term ethanol ingestion

S23.4 Which ONE of the following is *not* an indication for specialist referral in the context of a paracetamol overdose?

○ A Encephalopathy
○ B Prothrombin time the same as the control
○ C Hypoglycaemia
○ D Bicarbonate < 18 mmol/l
○ E Creatinine > 300 μmol/l

ANSWERS ON PAGES 190–191

Scenario 24

A 62-year-old patient is referred to the Emergency Department by her GP for progressive shortness of breath, recent haemoptysis and weight loss. Her past medical history is significant for COPD and type 2 diabetes, which is well controlled on metformin. She takes no other medications, takes occasional alcohol with her friends and stopped smoking 10 years ago, though smoked 40 a day for most of her adult life.

S24.1 What is the most useful initial investigation?

○ A D-Dimers
○ B CT chest
○ C Chest X-ray
○ D Transthoracic echocardiogram
○ E Bronchoscopy

Her blood results are returned as:

Haemoglobin	11.3 g/dl
MCV	80 fl
WCC	$10 \times 10^9/l$
Sodium	138 mmol/l
Potassium	4.2 mmol/l
Creatinine	170 µmol/l
Urea	12 mmol/l

Her renal function has been poor for a number of years but there appears to be no significant decline on this admission. Liver function tests and thyroid function tests are within normal limits. Blood sugars ranged from 10 to 15 mmol/l before and 15 to 20 mmol/l after eating. She has been booked for a CT scan of her chest.

42

ANSWER ON PAGE 192

S24.2 Which ONE of the following should be undertaken?

A 0.9% saline for 12 hours prior to the procedure

B Increase metformin to optimise her blood sugar control

C Check for metal implants

D ECG

E V/Q scan prior to procedure

questions

Scenario 25

A 52-year-old man is brought into the Emergency Department in severe abdominal pain. He reports going to a stag party and consuming in excess of 80 g of ethanol. The pain is epigastric and severe (10/10 in severity when questioned). It is associated with nausea and vomiting.

S25.1 Which ONE of the following is *not* a recognised cause of the above disease?

- ○ A Polyarteritis nodosa
- ○ B Hypothermia
- ○ C Endoscopic retrograde cholangiopancreatography
- ○ D Measles
- ○ E Hypertriglyceridaemia

S25.2 Which ONE of the following is *not* used in the assessment of severity in the above disease?

- ○ A Amylase
- ○ B Serum calcium
- ○ C Blood sugar
- ○ D Age
- ○ E White cell count

S25.3 Which ONE of the following statements about the above condition is true?

○ A Serum amylase is preferred over lipase in the diagnosis of the above condition

○ B The Glasgow score is valid 6 hours after presentation

○ C Enteral nutrition is of benefit in patients with the above condition

○ D Patients with persisting organ failure and severe disease will require serial abdominal X-rays to aid management

○ E If gallstones are suspected, ERCP should be delayed until clinical improvement occurs

questions

Scenario 26

A 52-year-old man is brought into the Emergency Department after suffering a fall secondary to alcohol intoxication. He is well known to the hospital, having had several admissions in the past year for similar alcohol-associated problems.

S26.1 Which ONE of the following agents is most commonly used for sedation in patients who undergo alcohol withdrawal?

○ A Diazepam

○ B Lorazepam

○ C Pabrinex

○ D Chlordiazepoxide

○ E Haloperidol

S26.2 Which ONE of the following is *not* commonly used in the treatment of alcohol withdrawal?

○ A Insulin

○ B Thiamine

○ C Pabrinex

○ D Intravenous phosphate

○ E Intravenous fluids

ANSWERS ON PAGE 195

S26.3 Which ONE of the following statements is *false*?

○   A   Subdural haematomas are more common in alcoholics

○   B   Delirium tremens occurs after 2–3 days of alcohol abstinence

○   C   Wernicke syndrome is the triad of ophthalmoplegia, nystagmus and amnesia

○   D   Acamprosate works by binding to NMDA receptors to increase abstinence to alcohol

○   E   Mortality of untreated delirium tremens is in the order of 30%

ANSWER ON PAGE 195

questions

Scenario 27

An 80-year-old patient is referred from a nursing home because of severe abdominal pain. On examination she in considerable discomfort with a distended abdomen and looks unwell. There is absolute constipation and the percussion note in resonant. Her recent past medical history is only significant for constipation.

S27.1 Which ONE of the following investigations is most useful initially?

- ○ A Abdominal X-ray
- ○ B Abdominal CT scan
- ○ C Endoscopy
- ○ D Ultrasound of the abdomen
- ○ E Cystoscopy

S27.2 Which ONE of the following is most likely?

- ○ A Bladder stone
- ○ B Sigmoid carcinoma
- ○ C Mesenteric ischaemia
- ○ D Sigmoid volvulus
- ○ E Perforated peptic ulcer

S27.3 Which ONE of the following is most useful in the above patient?

- ○ A Laparotomy
- ○ B Phosphate enema
- ○ C Gastrografin meal
- ○ D Flatus tube insertion
- ○ E Conservative management

ANSWERS ON PAGE 196

Scenario 28

A patient presents to the general practitioner with malaise and tiredness which have been present for a few weeks. She also complains of fevers, sweats and easy bruising but has not had frank bleeding. On examination the spleen is palpable 5 cm below the costal margin and there is 2-cm hepatomegaly. You organise urgent blood tests, which show a WCC of 125×10^9/l. You refer the patient to a consultant who performs further investigations, which show a t(9:22) translocation.

S28.1 What is the name given to the abnormality above?

○ A Amsterdam chromosome
○ B Hammersmith chromosome
○ C Philadelphia chromosome
○ D Cambridge chromosome
○ E Boston–Harvard chromosome

S28.2 What is the most likely diagnosis?

○ A Chronic myeloid leukaemia
○ B Chronic lymphocytic leukaemia
○ C Hodgkin's lymphoma
○ D Acute pro-myelocytic leukaemia
○ E Waldenström's macroglobulinaemia

S28.3 Which ONE of the following treatments is most suitable for this patient?

○ A Imatinib mesylate
○ B Hydroxyurea
○ C Bone marrow transplantation
○ D Ciclosporin
○ E Rituximab

49

Scenario 29

A 55-year-old patient presents with profound haematemesis. He looks very unwell and on examination has multiple spider naevi on his chest, gynaecomastia and a tender liver. A senior gastroenterology consultant is on his way to the endoscopy suite and in the meantime you have protected the patient's airway, established intravenous access, taken blood for haematology and clinical chemistry and started IV fluids.

S29.1 Which ONE of the following pharmacological agents should be given in the interim?

- A Propranolol
- B Vasopressin
- C Vitamin K
- D Dopamine
- E Terlipressin

The gastroenterology consultant manages to control the bleeding and the patient returns to the ward.

S29.2 Which ONE of the following should the patient be started on to prevent further episodes of bleeding?

- A Ramipril
- B Verapamil
- C Propranolol
- D Norfloxacin
- E Vasopressin

50

ANSWERS ON PAGE 198

SECTION 2:
KNOWLEDGE-BASED QUESTIONS

K1 **You are the F1 doctor attached to the diabetes team of your local hospital and are teaching the nursing staff about diabetic emergencies. Which ONE of the following statements is true?**

○ A Diabetic ketoacidosis only occurs in patients with type 1 diabetes mellitus

○ B The mortality rate of diabetic ketoacidosis is greater than that of hyperosmolar hyperglycaemic states

○ C Diabetic ketoacidosis typically has an onset of less than 24 hours

○ D A raised white cell count in a patient with diabetic ketoacidosis implies co-existent infection

○ E Under-dosing of insulin is the commonest factor precipitating diabetic ketoacidosis

K2   A 62-year-old man presents to the Emergency Department with acute-onset shortness of breath and haemoptysis. He had a hip replacement operation 2 weeks ago and has been finding the exercises to get him back on his feet very difficult. On examination he is tachypnoeic at rest, tachycardic with a pulse of 130/minute, has a pyrexia of 37.4 °C and oxygen saturations of 92% on room air.

Which ONE of the following is the most appropriate investigation in this patient?

- ○ A   Bronchoscopy
- ○ B   D-Dimer
- ○ C   ECG
- ○ D   Lateral chest X-ray
- ○ E   Blood cultures

K3   You are reviewing patients in the General Endocrine Clinic. Which ONE of the following statements is correct?

- ○ A   Prolactin is under positive feedback from dopamine released by the anterior pituitary
- ○ B   Cortisol secretion is diurnal, with levels being highest at midnight and lowest between 8 and 9am
- ○ C   In response to renal hypoperfusion the kidneys secrete angiotensin-converting enzyme, which converts angiotensinogen to angiotensin I
- ○ D   Aldosterone is secreted from the zona glomerulosa of the adrenal cortex and affects sodium and potassium homeostasis, particularly in the distal tubule of the kidney
- ○ E   LH stimulates the production of testosterone from Sertoli cells in the seminiferous tubule

K4 **You are the F1 doctor on call in the Medical Assessment Unit and are admitting Mrs Daisy Smith, a 92-year-old patient from a nearby nursing home for dehydration and a urinary tract infection. On examination you note a pressure sore over the sacrum. Which ONE of the following statements is MOST true?**

○ A Tissue viability nurse assessment is only required if surgical debridement is being considered

○ B A stage 4 pressure sore implies full-thickness skin loss with subcutaneous tissue involvement

○ C Confusion is a risk factor in the development of pressure sores

○ D Occlusive moist dressings such as hydrocolloid should be avoided

○ E Risk assessment should only be initiated in patients who you feel are likely to remain inpatients for more than 2 weeks

ANSWER ON PAGE 202

questions

K5 **A 24-year-old university student presents to her general practitioner with worsening tiredness and bruising. On examination she is extremely pale and has multiple bruises over her body. She is referred urgently to the local hospital, where a blood count shows:**

Haemoglobin	7.2 g/dl
WCC	2.08×10^9/l
Neutrophils	0.74×10^9/l
Platelets	48×10^9/l

She has no past medical history of note, takes no regular medications, and there is no significant family history apart from a distant aunt who has sickle cell disease. She does drink a few glasses of wine a week and smokes cigarettes occasionally but denies recreational drug use. She is reviewed by the haematologists, who perform a bone marrow biopsy which reveals a hypoplastic marrow.

Which ONE of the following is the most likely diagnosis?

- A Myelodysplastic syndrome
- B Aplastic anaemia
- C Evans syndrome
- D Myelofibrosis
- E Thrombotic thrombocytopenic purpura

ANSWER ON PAGE 203

K6 **A 22-year-old patient has a history of irregular menstrual cycles over the past few years. She is well known to you and has seen you regularly with regard to her weight problem, oily skin and acne. She presents to you on this occasion with a 5-month history of amenorrhoea and weight gain. Which ONE of the following is the most appropriate initial investigation in the above scenario?**

- A Pelvic ultrasound
- B Sex-hormone-binding globulin free androgen levels
- C LH:FSH levels
- D Oral glucose tolerance test
- E βhCG estimation

K7 **Which ONE of the following statements is true?**

- A Haemolytic disease of the newborn is caused by IgM antibodies
- B Goodpasture's disease is an example of a type III hypersensitivity reaction
- C Anaphylactic reactions are due to IgA antibodies
- D Red blood cells sensitised in vivo to autoantibodies can be detected using the direct Coombs' reaction
- E The human immunodeficiency virus uses CXCR4 and CCR5 a co-receptors to gain entry into CD8+ T cells

K8 **A 25-year-old patient presents with a 3-day history of a painful swollen knee, which has been getting progressively worse. He remembers falling over and banging his knee prior to the pain starting. He has never had a similar episode and does not see his general practitioner on a regular basis. He takes paracetamol occasionally for headaches which he suffers because of overwork but denies any other over-the-counter, alternative or illegal medication use. On examination his temperature is 38.5 °C, he is unable to move the knee and he looks unwell. What is the most important investigation to perform in this patient?**

○ A   Blood cultures

○ B   Clinically appropriate radiographs

○ C   Paracetamol levels

○ D   Aspiration of synovial fluid

○ E   Liver function tests

K9 **Which ONE of the following is a DNA virus?**

○ A   Hepatitis A virus

○ B   Hepatitis B virus

○ C   Hepatitis C virus

○ D   Measles virus

○ E   Mumps virus

ANSWERS ON PAGE 204

K10 **Which ONE of the following statements with regard to the electrocardiograph is correct?**

○ A ST depression and tall R waves in leads V1 and V2 is consistent with a diagnosis of a posterior myocardial infarction

○ B The corrected QT interval = QT interval / RR interval

○ C Obesity causes low-voltage QRS complexes

○ D 2-mm ST elevation in leads II, III, aVF, V4 and V5 is consistent with an inferior myocardial infarction

○ E S1Q3T3 is a common finding in patients diagnosed with a pulmonary embolism

K11 **Which ONE of the following statements is true?**

○ A The long saphenous vein runs from the sapheno-femoral junction to the medial malleolus

○ B The sapheno-femoral junction is 1 cm lateral and 1 cm inferior to the pubic tubercle

○ C The profunda femoris can be harvested and used as a replacement artery for coronary artery bypass grafting

○ D A saphena varix classically transmits a cough impulse and disappears when the patient is asked to stand up

○ E The Trendelenburg test is useful for assessing the competence of the sapheno-femoral junction

K12 A 60-year-old gentleman presents to the Emergency Department with sudden-onset severe central abdominal pain which is associated with vomiting and diarrhoea. He describes it as a constant pain that does not radiate and he has never had this pain before. His past medical history is significant for a myocardial infarction but he has not been diagnosed with any other problem. He does, however, report that he has recently experienced worsening heartburn after eating.

On examination he was initially extremely unwell with tachycardia and resistant hypotension despite aggressive fluid treatment. Abdominal examination revealed slight central and epigastric pain but no guarding or rebound tenderness.

Which ONE of the following is the most likely diagnosis?

○ A Perforated viscera

○ B Pancreatitis

○ C Gastric ulcer

○ D Small-bowel ischaemia

○ E Intussusception

K13 **Which ONE of the following statements is *not* part of the General Medical Council Duties of a Doctor?**

○ A Be honest and trustworthy

○ B Respect and protect confidential information at all times

○ C Recognise the limits of your professional competence

○ D Work with colleagues in a way which best serves the health service

○ E Give patients information in a way they can understand

ANSWERS ON PAGE 205

K14 **You are undertaking a placement in a family planning clinic during your general practice rotation. Which ONE of the following statements is true?**

○ A Condoms have a success rate of only 90%, even when used to their maximal effectiveness

○ B Failure rates of male surgical sterilisation are worse than for female surgical sterilisation

○ C The combined oral contraceptive pill can be used to treat acne vulgaris

○ D Breast cancer is not a contraindication for the use of the combined oral contraceptive pill

○ E Mrs Smith, a 35-year-old who smokes 20 cigarettes a day, can be safely started on the combined oral contraceptive pill

K15 **A 56-year-old lady presents with progressive tiredness, malaise and general apathy. She also states that her motions have been much looser recently and it is painful for her to eat. On examination she has difficulty appreciating sensation distally and a full blood count shows a haemoglobin of 9 g/dl and a MCV of 125 fl. Which ONE of the following is the most likely underlying diagnosis?**

○ A Hypothyroidism
○ B Hyperthyroidism
○ C Pernicious anaemia
○ D Addison's disease
○ E Carcinoma of the stomach

K16 You are an F1 doctor reviewing patients in the Dermatology Clinic. You are reviewing Mrs Jones, a 32-year-old patient originally from Australia who has had long-standing pompholyx affecting the fingers. During this attendance she says that her husband has noticed a new mole on her back which has been bleeding on contact. Which ONE of the following statements is true with regard to melanoma?

○ A Nodular melanoma is a highly aggressive form of the disease

○ B Superficial spreading melanoma, despite its name, usually exhibits vertical spread before lateral spread

○ C Clark's thickness represents the thickness of tumour depth

○ D Patients with metastatic disease have a 5-year survival of more than 50%

○ E Colour variegation should not raise suspicion as it is present in moles as well as melanoma

K17 A 52-year-old abattoir worker presents to the Emergency Department with a week-long history of shortness of breath, fevers and productive cough, which he describes as purulent with a rusty colour. He has recently returned from a week-long holiday with his friends in Spain, where he stayed in a large hotel. On examination he is pyrexial, with bronchial breathing at the right base. Which ONE of the following is the most likely diagnosis?

○ A *Coxiella burnetii*
○ B *Moraxella catarrhalis*
○ C *Legionella pneumophila*
○ D *Haemophilus influenzae*
○ E *Streptococcus pneumoniae*

ANSWERS ON PAGES 207–208

K18   **You are a junior doctor in the Emergency**
Department working the late shift and are
reviewing a known intravenous drug abuser
who is suspected to have bacterial endocarditis.
While taking blood cultures, you are slightly
distracted and accidentally stab your thumb on
the needle you used to take blood. Which ONE of
the following statements is true?

O   A   If the patient is HIV-positive the risk of contracting HIV
is 25%

O   B   There is a smaller risk of contracting HIV through a
needlestick injury than through exposure via mucous
membranes

O   C   Post-exposure prophylaxis is indicated in high-risk cases
only

O   D   The seroconversion rate for HIV is greater than for
hepatitis B following a needlestick injury

O   E   The doctor should finish taking blood before obtaining
treatment for himself

K19   **A worried parent brings her 15-year-old daughter to see you in general practice. The mother is concerned that her daughter is becoming increasingly thin and gaunt and has lost a considerable amount of weight after going on a crash diet. The patient feels that she is overweight and no amount of reasoning by her parents changes her beliefs. She has restricted the types and amounts of food she eats and exercises excessively. You calculate her weight to be 80% of predicted for her age, height and sex. Which ONE of the following is true with regard to the underlying diagnosis?**

- A   50 females are affected for every male affected
- B   Amenorrhoea often precedes weight loss
- C   The above diagnosis is more common in lower socioeconomic groups
- D   There is a marked increase in sexual activity
- E   In adults a body mass index (BMI) of less than 15 kg/m² is needed to confirm the diagnosis

ANSWER ON PAGE 209

K20 **With regard to consent, which ONE of the following is true?**

A A signed and dated consent form is evidence that valid consent has been obtained

B Capacity to give consent requires the patient to be able to read and write

C Provided you are working for the consultant undertaking the procedure, you are able to take valid consent for that procedure

D Only people with parental responsibility are allowed to give consent on behalf of children

E You are only required to inform patients of a complication if the complication rate is greater than 1%

K21 **Which ONE of the following statements about multiple sclerosis is true?**

A The commonest presentation of multiple sclerosis is primary progressive multiple sclerosis

B The lifetime risk of a sibling developing multiple sclerosis is not greater than that of the general population

C Normal optic discs imply a diagnosis other than optic neuritis in a patient with multiple sclerosis

D Oligoclonal bands in the CSF which match the serum are highly suggestive of multiple sclerosis

E Immobility is a contraindication to treatment with the disease-modifying beta-interferon medications

K22 **A 40-year-old woman who has been diagnosed with grand mal epilepsy was started on treatment after her second episode. You are the F2 in the Neurology Clinic and she meets you for the first time. She complains that her old shoes no longer fit and that her hair seems to have thinned over the past few months. She also complains that she is feeling more tired and has to take afternoon naps to keep going. On examination you note that she is slightly overweight and on direct questioning she admits her weight seems to have increased, although denies a change of diet. She also appears to have a mild tremor. Which ONE of the following is most likely in this patient?**

○ A The patient has an underlying pituitary disorder

○ B The features should raise suspicions of underlying depression

○ C The features are consistent with carbamazepine treatment

○ D The features are consistent with sodium valproate treatment

○ E The features are consistent with lamotrigine treatment

K23 **A 32-year-old housewife is referred to the Gastroenterology Clinic with a 2-year history of gastroenterological complaints. Which ONE of the following is most useful in her history in establishing an organic diagnosis?**

○ A Tenesmus

○ B Mucus per rectum

○ C Dyspareunia

○ D Abdominal bloating

○ E Weight loss

ANSWERS ON PAGE 212

K24 **Which ONE of the following is considered the gold-standard experimental study design to assess the relationship between two variables?**

○ A Systematic review
○ B Meta-analysis
○ C Cohort study
○ D Case–controlled study
○ E Randomised controlled trial

K25 **You are a final-year medical student in the Ophthalmology Clinic and have been asked to review a patient's optic discs and retina. Which ONE of the following agents should be used to dilate the patient's pupils?**

○ A Tropicamide
○ B Cyclopentolate
○ C Pilocarpine
○ D Adrenaline
○ E Tetracaine

K26 **Which ONE of the following diseases has the highest incidence of positive rheumatoid factor?**

○ A Sjögren syndrome
○ B Acute rheumatoid arthritis
○ C Systemic sclerosis
○ D Systemic lupus erythematosus
○ E Primary biliary cirrhosis

K27 **Cotton-wool calcification on a radiograph is classically associated with which ONE of the following conditions?**

A Osteosarcoma

B Ewing's sarcoma

C Chondrosarcoma

D Osteoclastoma

E Osteoid osteoma

K28 **Which ONE of the following is a Schneiderian first-rank symptom?**

A Visual hallucinations

B Delusional perceptions

C Olfactory hallucinations

D Déjà vu

E Thought block

K29 **Which ONE of the following matches the correct visual defect with the correct lesion?**

A Bitemporal hemianopia – occipital cortex

B Right superior homonymous quadrantanopia – left parietal cortex

C Left homonymous scotoma – right occipital cortex

D Left inferior homonymous quadrantanopia – right temporal cortex

E Right monocular anopia – right occipital cortex

K30 A 53-year-old male engineer has returned from the United Arab Emirates where he was working in the desert for a number of years on a new construction project. He comes to you in the clinic with a growth on his left eye. On examination a greyish-yellow nodule is noted which extends onto the cornea in a wedge-shaped manner. What is the most likely diagnosis?

- A Squamous cell carcinoma
- B Hordeolum internum
- C Pinguecula
- D Pterygium
- E Hordeolum externum

K31 In which ONE of the following conditions is the Köbner phenomenon *least* likely to be seen?

- A Vitiligo
- B Pityriasis rosea
- C Warts
- D Lichen planus
- E Psoriasis

K32 A patient presents acutely with a red eye and is in a significant amount of pain, with a marked degree of photophobia. The patient also describes blurred vision and floaters. Which ONE of the following is most likely in the above patient?

- A Viral conjunctivitis
- B Bacterial conjunctivitis
- C Open angle glaucoma
- D Closed angle glaucoma
- E Uveitis

ANSWERS ON PAGE 214

K33 **A 34-year-old lady presents in your general practice surgery with a history of worsening hearing and tinnitus. She is currently pregnant and her hearing has deteriorated significantly but you note her hearing problems were present prior to her pregnancy as well. Her father and grandfather both suffered from poor hearing and she is worried about the future. Which ONE of the following statements is true?**

A She should be reassured that the hearing loss is transient and that her hearing will return to normal with the delivery of the baby

B She should be told to avoid areas with background noise as this will make her hearing worse

C The condition is due to ankylosis

D Surgical treatment of this condition leads to deafness in 1/1000 people who undergo the operation

E Audiometry in this patient would show a marked dip at 8 kHz

K34 **A female patient attends the Emergency Department because of worsening shortness of breath which is associated with worsening rhinitis and sinusitis. On examination she has a lesion of the facial nerve on the right. Blood tests showed a markedly raised eosinophil count with raised ESR. She says that her GP sent her for a chest X-ray in the past for similar symptoms and it was reported as abnormal. Which ONE of the following is most likely?**

A Allergic asthma

B Polyarteritis nodosa

C Infective exacerbation of asthma

D Churg–Strauss syndrome

E SLE

K35 **In which ONE of the following conditions are you most likely to hear wide fixed splitting of the second heart sound on auscultation?**

○ A Right bundle branch block
○ B Atrial septal defect
○ C Ventricular septal defect
○ D Left bundle branch block
○ E Patent ductus arteriosus

K36 **Which ONE of the following areas is assessed in the Barthel score?**

○ A Shopping
○ B Coordination
○ C Cooking
○ D Stability
○ E Toilet use

K37 **You are the F1 doctor in cardiology and are reviewing the drug charts of your patients. Which ONE of the following statements is true?**

○ A Loop diuretics exert their effects by acting on sodium/potassium/bicarbonate channels in the thick ascending limb of the loop of Henle

○ B Amiloride promotes potassium reabsorption in the collecting duct, accounting for its potassium-sparing effects

○ C Metolazone is a powerful thiazide diuretic used in patients with severe and resistant heart failure

○ D Flecainide is the agent of choice in patients with atrial fibrillation and a background of coronary heart disease

○ E Patients on amiodarone should have regular check-ups of their thyroid and renal function

K38 **Which ONE of the following statements is true with regard to delirium?**

○   A   Confusion tends to get better as the day progresses

○   B   Sensory deprivation is a risk factor for the development of delirium

○   C   Visual hallucinations are suggestive of an alternative diagnosis

○   D   Haloperidol is absolutely contraindicated in the management of delirium

○   E   The vast majority of patients with delirium have underlying dementia

K39 **Which ONE of the following statements with regard to Salter–Harris fractures is true?**

○   A   Type III fractures are the most common

○   B   They can occur at any age

○   C   They are more common in girls

○   D   The Salter–Harris classification system includes greenstick fractures

○   E   The type V fracture is a crush fracture

K40 **Which ONE of the following statements is true with regard to immunisation?**

○   A   The diphtheria, tetanus and polio vaccines are recommended to be given eight times between birth and the age of 18 years

○   B   There has been an increased incidence of measles due to the link between MMR and autism

○   C   Herd immunity plays a minimal role in protecting the community

○   D   The tetanus vaccine is a toxin-based vaccine

○   E   The BCG vaccine is an attenuated strain of *Mycobacterium tuberculosis*

K41 A 64-year-old lady is admitted with severe pneumonia with consolidation seen on her chest X-ray. While on the ward she develops a warm, erythematous, tender and oedematous left leg. A few days later, her breathing, which was improving with antibiotic treatment suddenly deteriorates. Which ONE of the following is *least* useful in the above patient?

○ A Pulse

○ B Blood pressure

○ C CT pulmonary angiogram

○ D V/Q scan

○ E Arterial blood gas measurement

K42 A 78-year-old woman develops left-sided chest pain and tingling. This is the first episode of this type of pain and is not associated with any shortness of breath, dizziness, nausea or vomiting. She is a lifelong smoker and takes simvastatin for hypercholesterolaemia. On placing the ECG electrodes on the chest you notice a band-like area of erythema on the left side of her chest. The ECG you carry out shows left ventricular hypertrophy and non-specific T-wave changes. Which ONE of the following options best applies to this patient?

○ A Start antiviral therapy

○ B Admit the patient to the Coronary Care Unit

○ C Give ibuprofen for the pain

○ D Measure troponin levels

○ E Perform a transthoracic echocardiogram

K43   A 55-year-old patient is referred by his general practitioner to the General Surgery Clinic at the local hospital because of a left varicocoele and haematuria. On examination the patient has an abdominal mass on the left-hand side. A chest X-ray shows multiple coin lesions in both lung fields. Which ONE of the following is the most likely diagnosis?

○   A   Transitional cell carcinoma

○   B   Renal cell carcinoma

○   C   Seminoma

○   D   Prostate carcinoma

○   E   Teratoma

K44   A 72-year-old gentleman who is known to suffer from dementia develops a urinary tract infection that requires admission to hospital. He is on the ward for a few days and seems to be improving with oral antibiotic treatment. You get a call from the nurse in charge informing you that he has deteriorated and ask the medical student under your supervision to go and take a history and perform an examination. The medical student reports that over the past day he seems to have been getting more confused and that it was not possible to take a history. His pulse, blood pressure and respiratory rate are stable. She states that the abdomen seems more distended and thinks she can feel a mass in the lower abdomen with dullness to percussion. What is the ONE most appropriate diagnostic step?

○   A   Arrange for a CT scan of the abdomen

○   B   Take blood for full blood count, urea and electrolytes and CRP

○   C   Arrange for urgent catheterisation

○   D   Arrange for an urgent ultrasound of the abdomen

○   E   Urine analysis to assess for infection

K45 A 45-year-old patient presents to you with a few weeks' history of odynophagia and dysphagia. On examination he is noted to have white plaques at the back of his throat although no ulcers can be seen. On endoscopy these white plaques extend into the oesophagus. He does not take any prescription drugs, over-the-counter remedies or illegal drugs. There is nothing of note in his past medical history. What is the SINGLE most useful test in diagnosing the *underlying* pathology in this patient?

○ A Monospot test
○ B Oral glucose tolerance test
○ C Blood tests
○ D Viral markers
○ E Bacterial microscopy, culture and sensitivity

K46 A young child in brought to you by her worried mother with an erythematous rash on her cheeks but is otherwise well. On examination she has a slapped-cheek appearance. Which ONE of the following is the most likely organism responsible?

○ A Human herpesvirus 6
○ B Parvovirus B19
○ C *Staphylococcus aureus*
○ D Beta-haemolytic *Streptococcus*
○ E Measles virus

questions

K47   Which ONE of the following statements related to pregnancy and conception is true?

O   A   Haemoglobin levels rise in pregnancy

O   B   Both ventilation and depth of breathing decrease

O   C   Cardiac output increases due to increased pulse but not stroke volume

O   D   Maternal cortisol output decreases although free levels remain fairly constant

O   E   The pregnancy test is usually positive 2 weeks after conception, not the last menstrual period

K48   You are an F2 doctor assisting your consultant in his thyroid clinic, which ONE of the following is true?

O   A   A patient who has been diagnosed with hypothyroidism and started on 50 micrograms of thyroxine should have their thyroid function measured every 2–3 weeks to assess the response

O   B   In Graves' disease the stimulating antibodies exert their effects on the parafollicular cells within the thyroid gland

O   C   Carbimazole exerts its effects by inhibiting the release of preformed thyroxine from the thyroid gland

O   D   The majority of cold nodules seen on nuclear imaging of the thyroid are benign

O   E   Follicular carcinoma is the commonest type of thyroid malignancy

ANSWERS ON PAGES 221–222

K49   A 60-year-old police officer presents with pain in his left knee, which seems to getting worse over the past year. On radiography there is a distinct opaque line that is in keeping with calcification in the menisci. Which ONE of the following is true with regard to this condition?

○   A   Synovial fluid examination would reveal needle-shaped crystals that are negatively birefringent in polarised light

○   B   The condition shows two peaks in incidence with respect to age

○   C   Progression of the disease would see punched-out lesions in juxta-articular bone

○   D   Hyperparathyroidism increases the risk of developing the condition

○   E   The condition is typically associated with rheumatoid arthritis

K50   A 20-year-old male athlete presents to you with increasing back pain and morning stiffness which lasts for a few hours. He also reports that he has been having considerable difficulty reaching his toes when warming up for his exercises. Which ONE of the following is true about this disease?

○   A   The disease is associated with HLA-B21

○   B   The disease typically shows evidence of an IgM antibody directed against the Fc portion of immunoglobulins

○   C   The disease is associated with valvular heart disease

○   D   Patients have a higher risk of developing AL amyloidosis

○   E   Infliximab has been shown to be ineffective in the treatment of the disease

K51 **A 25-year-old single mother presents with a breast lump. This is the first time she has noticed such a lump and is worried because her mother died of breast cancer at the age of 50. On examination she appears well and the lump is smooth, approximately 2 cm in diameter, freely mobile and not fixed to skin or underlying muscle. On examination of the axilla you cannot palpate any masses. What is the most likely diagnosis?**

○ A Fibroadenoma

○ B Fat necrosis

○ C Fibrocystic disease

○ D Carcinoma in situ

○ E Breast cyst

K52 **A 15-year-old boy presents with a rash on his buttocks, arms and legs, a few days after a sore throat. The mother is extremely worried because on trying the tumbler test, the rash did not go away. He also complains of pain in his joints and abdomen and urine dipstick shows the presence of blood and protein. What is the most likely diagnosis?**

○ A Disseminated bacterial meningitis

○ B Haemolytic uraemic syndrome

○ C Disseminated intravascular coagulation

○ D Goodpasture's disease

○ E Henoch–Schönlein purpura

ANSWERS ON PAGE 223

K53 A 70-year-old man has come to see you with fullness in the abdomen and tiredness. His health has generally been very good and he reports no problems apart from a few lumps that appear occasionally but slowly subside. His routine blood tests show anaemia, with a decrease in the haptoglobin levels and a marked lymphocytosis. What is the most likely diagnosis?

A   Chronic lymphocytic leukaemia
B   Acute lymphocytic leukaemia
C   Acute pro-myelocytic leukaemia
D   Hodgkin's disease
E   Multiple myeloma

K54 A 45-year-old clerical assistant comes to see you in general practice with a sore throat that has been getting worse over the last week and which is really affecting her work. She also reports a non-productive cough which she has had for the last 2 weeks and that she is feeling hot and bothered. Her medical history is significant for treated hyperthyroidism and vitiligo, for which she has been seen by a dermatologist. Which ONE the following is the most appropriate?

A   Send the patient for an urgent chest X-ray
B   Request urgent thyroid function tests
C   Request an urgent full blood count
D   Request a monospot test
E   Start the patient on steroids and amoxicillin

questions

questions

K55 **Which ONE of the following is *not* typically inherited in an autosomal recessive manner?**

○ A Hereditary haemochromatosis

○ B Hereditary spherocytosis

○ C Wilson's disease

○ D Infantile polycystic kidney disease

○ E Cystic fibrosis

K56 **A 92-year-old gentleman is brought into the Emergency Department with dehydration and continual vomiting. He is known to have a large caecal adenocarcinoma but has been deemed too high an operative risk by the surgeons, who are unwilling to operate. You start intravenous fluids and insert a large-bore nasogastric (NG) tube, which relieves some of his symptoms. After 5 days he continues to deteriorate, with worsening abdominal tenderness and large volumes of NG aspirate. After discussion with the family and taking into account the patient's wishes it is decided to keep the patient comfortable and start him on the Liverpool Care Pathway for the dying patient. Which ONE of the following statements is true with regard to end-of-life care?**

○ A The Liverpool Care Pathway should only be used when cancer is the underlying diagnosis

○ B Fluids are routinely continued to prevent dehydration in the dying patient

○ C Octreotide has a useful role in the above patient

○ D Metoclopramide would be a useful subcutaneous antiemetic in the above patient

○ E Medication should be given on a p.r.n. basis as much as possible to avoid distress caused by a continuous syringe driver infusion

ANSWERS ON PAGES 224–225

K57 **A patient is brought into the Emergency Department short of breath and in chest pain. On ECG testing there is a rate of 175/minute which is regular, while the QRS distance measures 0.08 seconds. He is currently haemodynamically stable and although the Valsava manoeuvre was attempted it did not affect the heart rate or rhythm. Which ONE of the following should be used next?**

- O A Amiodarone
- O B Atropine
- O C Vagal manoeuvres
- O D Digoxin
- O E Adenosine

K58 **You are an accident and emergency officer and a 60-year-old lady is brought in by the police after she was seen to be acting strangely in the street. She has wild, flinging movements of her arms. She has had multiple transient ischaemic attacks in the past. Which part of the brain is most likely to be affected?**

- O A Corpus callosum
- O B Subthalamic nucleus
- O C Superior temporal gyrus
- O D Midbrain
- O E Posterior inferior cerebellum

ANSWERS ON PAGE 225

K59 **Which ONE of the following is *least* likely to cause pruritis ani?**

○ A Threadworm

○ B Incontinence

○ C Anxiety

○ D Perianal haematoma

○ E Contact dermatitis

K60 **Which ONE of the following is in keeping with a tumour within the cerebellopontine angle?**

○ A Contralateral cerebellar signs

○ B Diminished corneal reflex

○ C 'Down and out' pupil

○ D Ipsilateral sternocleidomastoid weakness

○ E Myotonic pupil

K61 **A 45-year-old usually fit and active patient presents with acute pain in his right calf, from the knee downwards, causing him great difficulty in walking. On examination pulses are not palpable on the right below the knee. While standing the right limb appears more erythematous than the left, but this colour quickly fades on laying the patient flat. Which ONE of the following statements is *incorrect*?**

○ A Chronic arterial insufficiency is a likely underlying factor in this patient

○ B Sensation would also be decreased

○ C Ankle-brachial pressure index measurement is of limited use in this patient

○ D A Fogarty catheter can be used to treat this condition

○ E Sympathectomy is not indicated in this condition

ANSWERS ON PAGE 226

K62 **You are the F2 on call and the registrar asks you to comment on the CSF results of a patient in the Emergency Department:**

Blood glucose	6 mmol/l
Blood total protein	60 g/l
CSF cell count	357/mm^3
CSF glucose	4 mmol/l
CSF protein	0.78 g/l
CSF microscopy and culture	Investigation pending

Which statement best fits with the above results?

○ A The results are suggestive of viral meningitis

○ B You cannot comment on the results until the microscopy and culture has been completed

○ C The most likely cells to be seen are polymorphonuclear cells

○ D The results indicate that urgent antituberculous treatment should be initiated

○ E The results are in keeping with a parasitic infection

K63 **You are an F1 in general practice and are being consulted by Mrs Shah, who presents with a 3-month history of tiredness. She saw the GP principal previously who requested a full blood count. The results are shown below:**

Haemoglobin	9 g/dl
MCV	70 fl
Platelets	268×10^9/l
White cell differential	Normal

Which is the condition *least* likely to lead to the above?

- A Lead poisoning
- B Thalassaemia
- C Anaemia of chronic disease
- D Hypothyroidism
- E Sideroblastic anaemia

K64 **You are reviewing a 55-year-old patient referred by the general practitioner in the Rheumatology Clinic. He gives a month-long history of worsening arthralgia associated with deep ulcers over the feet which are not responding to oral antibiotic treatment. This has been associated with new-onset Raynaud's phenomenon and a purpuric rash on his shins. Urine dipstick shows the presence of blood and protein. His past medical history is significant for viral hepatitis. Which ONE of the following is the most likely diagnosis?**

- A Henoch–Schönlein purpura
- B Membranous glomerulonephritis
- C Cryoglobulinaemia
- D Haemolytic uraemic syndrome
- E Systemic lupus erythematosus

ANSWERS ON PAGES 227–228

K65 **Which ONE of the following is a notifiable disease?**

O A Syphilis
O B Hepatitis A
O C Human immunodeficiency virus
O D Traveller's diarrhoea
O E Influenza

K66 **A 70-year-old is brought into the Emergency Department with severe abdominal pain which has been getting worse over the past 2 days and has been associated with a fever at home. He reports that he has had some bloody diarrhoea at the same time. He attended a birthday party at a Chinese restaurant a few days ago and has been feeling unwell since then.**

On examination he is febrile, tachycardic and in obvious discomfort. Examination of his abdomen reveals a tender mass in the left iliac fossa with a degree of guarding. Rectal examination reveals normal-coloured stool with some blood on the glove but no evidence of melaena or masses. An erect chest X-ray does not show any evidence of subdiaphragmatic air.

Which ONE of the following is the most likely diagnosis?

O A Infective colitis
O B Ulcerative colitis
O C Malignant obstruction
O D Diverticulitis
O E Atypical appendicitis

83

K67 **A patient with mild seasonal asthma is brought in with severe breathlessness. You sit the patient upright and ask for her name and address and about what happened. You learn from her that she is called Lisa, a 24-year-old sales assistant working at the fashion counter in Harrods. She also complains of tingling in her arms. You start her on high-flow oxygen and someone hands you the results of her arterial blood gas analysis, which are shown below:**

pH	7.50
PaO$_2$	12.2 kPa
PaCO$_2$	3.1 kPa
Bicarbonate	30 mmol/l

What is the most appropriate next step?

○ A The results do not fit the clinical scenario, so repeat the arterial blood gas analysis

○ B The results are suggestive of a venous sample and should be repeated

○ C The anaesthetist should be notified and the patient intubated immediately

○ D The patient should be given supportive care

○ E The patient should be given nebulised salbutamol, ipratropium and intravenous steroids

ANSWER ON PAGE 229

K68 A 65-year-old man brings his partner into the general practice clinic because he has 'become a different person'. It is obvious when the patient walks through the door that he has difficulty walking, with a broad-based, shuffling gait. However, when the patient sits down you cannot elicit any evidence of slowness or rigidity. You also learn that he has been having trouble getting to the toilet in time to pass water and has also been forgetting his way around the house. Which ONE of the following diagnoses bests fits with this scenario?

○ A Parkinson's disease

○ B Alzheimer's disease

○ C Lewy body dementia

○ D Normal-pressure hydrocephalus

○ E Neurosyphilis

K69 Which ONE of the following is *not* an indication for urgent dialysis?

○ A Hyperkalaemia

○ B Significant uraemia

○ C Furosemide-resistant fluid overload

○ D Uraemic pericarditis

○ E Alkalosis

K70 **A 54-year-old accountant comes to see you because he has started coughing up blood. He is a lifelong heavy smoker and today he looks pale and he tells you he has become increasingly breathless, tired and weak over the past few months. Blood tests show his calcium to be elevated but he has no bony pain. Investigations reveal a malignancy with no metastatic disease evident. Which ONE of the following is the most likely diagnosis?**

    A Squamous cell carcinoma

    B Adenocarcinoma

    C Carcinoid tumour

    D Oat cell tumour

    E Alveolar cell carcinoma

K71 **A 29-year-old advertising executive develops nausea, vomiting and diarrhoea, which appears to be due to gastroenteritis. It later emerges that nearly everyone who attended the same conference 2 days ago has developed the same condition. Which ONE of the following applies to this patient?**

    A You do not need to contact the consultant in communicable disease

    B The timing is suggestive of *Salmonella* gastroenteritis

    C Antimicrobial therapy is the main treatment option in this patient

    D The pathogen is likely to be *Campylobacter jejuni*

    E The pathogen is likely to be *Bacillus cereus*

ANSWERS ON PAGE 229

K72 A 57-year-old gentleman presents with central chest pain with associated lower jaw pain while running for the bus. The pain lasted for half an hour and he describes it as a central stabbing pain and a dull ache with associated shortness of breath. He works as a computer programmer and recently flew back from America, where he was at a conference. He is otherwise well and is an ex-smoker, giving up 10 years ago, and drinks alcohol in moderation. He does say that there is family history of heart and lung problems: two of his brothers have had stents put into their heart and one of his sisters developed a clot in her leg during her pregnancy. The ECG shows some T-wave inversion in the lateral leads but no ST-segment abnormalities. A blood test 12 hours after the initial pain is returned as normal. Which ONE of the following is the most appropriate investigation based on these features?

- A Coronary angiogram
- B D-Dimer blood test
- C CT pulmonary angiogram
- D Discharge
- E Exercise tolerance test

K73 A 5-year-old asylum seeker from Africa is brought to see you in the Surgical Outpatient Clinic. You notice that he has a mass arising from the side of the neck, anterior to the sternocleidomastoid, which transilluminates brightly. What is the most likely diagnosis from the list below?

- A Laryngocoele
- B Cervical rib
- C Cystic hygroma
- D Branchial cysts
- E None of the above

K74 **Which ONE of the following statements best describes Charcot's triad?**

A Pain, dilated common bile duct and jaundice

B Pain, jaundice and fever

C Gallstones, pain and fever

D Gallstones, jaundice and hypoalbuminaemia

E Hypoalbuminaemia, pain and jaundice

K75 **A firefighter was brought into the Emergency Department after suffering major burns to his body while tackling a fire. The front of both of his legs, the front of his chest and abdomen and his entire right arm suffered significant burns. What is the approximate area of burns in this patient?**

A 36%

B 45%

C 54%

D 63%

E 72%

K76 **You are admitting an elderly gentleman from a nursing home who has been referred with increasing confusion secondary to a presumed urinary tract infection. On examination you hear an ejection systolic murmur which you think might be a sign of aortic stenosis. Which ONE of the following indicates severe aortic stenosis?**

A Grade 6 murmur

B Collapsing pulse

C Soft second heart sound

D Left ventricular hypertrophy on ECG

E Valve area of 2 cm^2

ANSWERS ON PAGES 230–231

K77 **A patient is brought into the Emergency Department acutely confused and in an agitated state, swearing and shouting abuse at both staff and other patients. On limited examination it is obvious he has a chest infection, which requires treatment and admission, and he is started on a number of medications. On review later the patient appears to be extremely sweaty, warm to touch and on attempting to move his arms he is very stiff. His pulse is 120/minute and blood pressure 90/60 mmHg. Which ONE of the following is most likely to cause these symptoms?**

- A Benzylpenicillin
- B Ceftriaxone
- C Haloperidol
- D Metoclopramide
- E Procyclidine

K78 **A 45-year-old solicitor is in a nightclub and experiences a very severe occipital headache, which he describes as the worst headache ever. He is brought into the Emergency Department within 2 hours of the headache and a CT scan is performed, which shows no abnormality. He is currently stable with a GCS score of 15/15. Which ONE of the following is the most suitable next step in this patient?**

- A Immediate lumbar puncture
- B Angiography
- C MRI scan
- D Supportive management
- E Ultrasound of the abdomen

K79 **A 68-year-old patient presents with recurrent haematuria which has been getting progressively worse over the past 2 weeks. He reports no pain or other urinary symptoms. Which diagnosis should be considered *first* in this patient?**

○ A Bladder stone

○ B Transitional cell carcinoma

○ C Squamous cell carcinoma

○ D Renal cell carcinoma

○ E Enterovesical fistula

K80 **A 24-year-old patient first came to see you in the general practice clinic because her home pregnancy test was positive. Following her through her pregnancy you always felt her uterus was much larger for dates than expected. She also needed hospitalisation and fluid rehydration for hyperemesis gravidarum. Your clinical suspicion was confirmed when she attends for her ultrasound. Which ONE of the following is *least* likely to complicate the above pregnancy?**

○ A Oligohydramnios

○ B Anaemia

○ C Pre-eclampsia

○ D Placenta praevia

○ E Placental abruption

ANSWERS ON PAGES 232–233

K81 **You are the F1 doctor in the Urology Department and insert a urinary catheter into an 82-year-old gentleman with urinary retention secondary to prostatic disease. You manage to perform the procedure but with great difficulty. You get bleeped to return to the ward by the nurses because the patient is complaining of severe discomfort at the front of his penis. Which statement is most likely to be true?**

O A The catheter was inserted without any local anaesthetic
O B The catheter that was inserted was too large
O C The patient is suffering from phimosis
O D The patient is suffering from paraphimosis
O E The catheter is irritating his bladder and causing referred pain

K82 **A patient is involved in a road traffic accident and is brought into the Emergency Department. On examination the right leg appears shortened, lies adducted, and is internally rotated and slightly flexed. Which ONE of the following bests fits with the above appearance?**

O A Fractured neck of femur
O B Anterior dislocation of the hip
O C Posterior dislocation of the hip
O D Fractured pelvic rami
O E Fractured mid-shaft of femur

K83 **Which ONE of the following statements is true with regard to rheumatoid arthritis?**

○ A Patients with the condition are at increased risk of developing coronary heart disease

○ B A swan-neck deformity is due to hyperflexion at the proximal interphalangeal joint

○ C Felty syndrome is the association of this disease with neutropenia and hepatomegaly

○ D Joints damaged by rheumatoid arthritis typically show a pencil-in-cup appearance

○ E The disease is associated with HLA-DQ1

K84 **Which ONE of the following dermatomes is most likely to provide sensation over the middle toe on the left side?**

○ A S1
○ B L5
○ C L4
○ D L3
○ E L2

K85   It is a Friday night and you are working as an F2 in the Emergency Department. At 1am a patron at a local pub is brought in after being involved in a fight. He smells strongly of alcohol and has numerous cuts and bruises over his face. When you ask him his name you get no response but he starts shouting obscenities when you apply pressure over his sternum. At the same time he opens his eyes and uses his other hand to push your hand away from his chest. What is the patient's Glasgow Coma Scale score?

○   A   6
○   B   7
○   C   9
○   D   10
○   E   11

K86   A 55-year-old patient with severe rheumatoid arthritis is admitted for an elective operation on her hands to help her functioning. She is a lifelong smoker of 5 cigarettes a day and reports a long-standing cough, she had a chest X-ray taken 2 months ago. She takes NSAIDs for pain and is on steroids to control her rheumatoid arthritis. You are responsible for making sure she is fit for surgery. Which ONE of the following measures is the most appropriate in this patient?

○   A   Neck X-ray
○   B   Full blood count
○   C   Repeat chest X-ray
○   D   Stop steroids before operation
○   E   Endoscopy

K87 **Which ONE of the following statements with regard to the Mental Health Act is true?**

O A The Emergency Department is counted as a hospital ward

O B A Section 3 is to enable treatment to be given and lasts for 6 months longer than a Section 2

O C Should police officers feel an individual is suffering from a mental illness in a public place, a Section 135 allows them to bring that individual to medical attention and a place of safety

O D Patients suffering from borderline personality disorder can be sectioned for assessment and treatment

O E A Section 4 is used for emergency detention of a patient already in the hospital

K88 **Listed below are a number of familial cancer syndromes. Which ONE has a different mode of inheritance compared with the others?**

O A Xeroderma pigmentosa

O B Familial breast cancer

O C Familial adenomatous polyposis

O D Hereditary non-polyposis colon cancer

O E Wilms' tumour

ANSWERS ON PAGE 235

K89 **A patient in hospital develops constipation during his admission and asks you, the F1 in charge of his care, about the medications available for this condition. Which statement is most correct from the list below?**

○ A Fybogel is a stimulant laxative which should be taken with plenty of fluids

○ B Magnesium-containing antacids can relieve constipation

○ C Lactulose is an stimulant laxative that can take up to 2 days to work

○ D Co-danthramer is a widely used stimulant laxative

○ E Hyperkalaemia is a risk with excessive use of laxatives

K90 **A 70-year-old patient presents to you with worsening backache for which you perform some blood tests. They are returned showing a raised ESR and hypercalcaemia. You arrange for urine electrophoresis, which proves the diagnosis. Which ONE of the following statements is most correct?**

○ A Alkaline phosphatase is usually raised in this condition

○ B Punched-out lesions on X-rays would be more in keeping with Paget's disease

○ C Urine electrophoresis detects the cell causing this condition

○ D Bone lesions in this disease are typically sclerotic

○ E Levels of a subunit of the MHC class I unit provides useful prognostic information

K91 **A 28-year-old man presents with increasing weakness of his legs and arms that has been getting worse over the past week. On examination, weakness can be demonstrated which is worse in the legs compared with the upper body, with absent reflexes bilaterally. He mentions that he had food poisoning recently but was fit and well apart from that. He takes no regular medications. Which ONE of the following is the most useful investigation in the above condition?**

A MRI spine

B Therapeutic trial with high-dose steroids

C EMG studies

D Spirometry

E Blood film

K92 **A 54-year-old patient complains of increasing difficulty swallowing over the past year. She reports no weight loss or sinister features suggestive of malignancy, but does say the food sticks in her throat. Which ONE of the following would you perform first to investigate this complaint?**

A Endoscopy

B Simple barium meal

C Barium swallow

D Double-contrast barium meal

E Small-bowel follow-through

K93 **Reed–Sternberg cells are the hallmark of which disease?**

○ A Hodgkin's lymphoma
○ B Non-Hodgkin's lymphoma
○ C Acute myeloid leukaemia
○ D Chronic myeloid leukaemia
○ E Chronic lymphocytic leukaemia

K94 **In order to review the complications that arise when patients receive blood or blood products a reporting system is in place in the UK. Which ONE of the following is the correct reporting system?**

○ A PILOT
○ B TRANSFUSE
○ C SHOT
○ D BSHRS
○ E GOLD

K95 **A 40-year-old patient comes to you with palpitations, weight loss and difficulty cooling down, even in winter. On examination of his eyes the white of the sclera was noted to be visible above and below the pupil, with lid lag. Which ONE of the following tests is most useful in this patient?**

○ A Thyroid-stimulating hormone
○ B Thyroid microsomal antibodies
○ C Thyroglobulin levels
○ D Thyroid-releasing hormone
○ E Free T4 levels

questions

K96 **A 76-year-old retired shop assistant who now lives in nursing home complains of pain in her chest along with haemoptysis. She is a lifelong non-smoker and denies any other illnesses, although she is just recovering from influenza. On examination she is febrile, uncomfortable at rest, with definite signs of consolidation on examination of the chest. Chest X-ray reveals consolidation of the upper lobes with cavitation. Which ONE of the following is the most likely organism?**

- A *Mycobacterium tuberculosis*
- B *Klebsiella pneumoniae*
- C *Legionella pneumoniae*
- D *Mycoplasma pneumoniae*
- E *Staphylococcus aureus*

K97 **Which ONE of the following is *not* part of clinical governance?**

- A Participating in clinical audit to improve services and processes
- B Teaching undergraduate medical students to further improve medical knowledge
- C Ensuring staff are immunised against infectious diseases
- D Ensuring current guidelines and evidence-based recommendations from research are implemented quickly and efficiently
- E Discussing performance of individuals or groups and established processes in an open and impartial way

ANSWERS ON PAGE 237

K98 You review a patient in the Gastroenterology Clinic with a diagnosed oesophageal stricture. Which ONE of the following is the most common cause of oesophageal strictures?

○ A Adenocarcinoma

○ B Crohn's disease

○ C Gastro-oesophageal reflux disease

○ D Caustic ingestion

○ E Radiation-induced stricture

K99 A patient presents to you with discomfort in his legs that has been getting progressively worse and is interfering with his sleep. He says that at night his legs become troublesome and he has to move them to get relief, commonly by pacing up and down the room. The discomfort is worse at rest and is associated with pins and needles or a crawling sensation. He is on no regular medication and has no significant medical history. Which ONE of the following is the most likely diagnosis?

○ A Femoral nerve entrapment

○ B Ekbom syndrome

○ C Arterial insufficiency

○ D Nocturnal leg cramps

○ E Akathisia

questions

K100 **A 52-year-old type 2 diabetic is seen by her general practitioner complaining of swollen legs and shortness of breath on exertion which has got much worse recently. On examination there are crackles at both bases with pitting oedema to the knee bilaterally. On further questioning she says that she was recently seen in the hospital Diabetes Clinic and that her medication was changed. Which ONE of the following is the most likely cause of her symptoms?**

    A Gliclazide

    B Metformin

    C Acarbose

    D Glargine

    E Rosiglitazone

K101 **A 55-year-old gentleman presents with paroxysmal nocturnal dyspnoea, three-pillow orthopnoea and crackles at the bases of his lungs. While further investigations are being organised you organise a full blood count, which reveals a raised MCV. What is the most likely diagnosis in this patient?**

    A Infective endocarditis

    B Hypertensive heart failure

    C Dilated cardiomyopathy

    D Ischaemic heart disease

    E Pericarditis

ANSWERS ON PAGE 238

K102 **A 25-year-old patient presents to the Sexual Health Clinic complaining of strange lesions in the anal region. They do not cause him any pain or discomfort but have been noticed by his partner recently. On examination there are numerous lesions, which are well circumscribed and have a pearly-white appearance. Some of them express a curd-like substance. Which ONE of the following is most likely to be responsible?**

- A Rhabdovirus
- B Herpesvirus
- C Papovavirus
- D Poxvirus
- E Adenovirus

K103 **A 62-year-old gentleman is admitted from the Emergency Department with shortness of breath. He is brought to the ward after stabilisation and you are the F1 on call. The nurses bleep you because he is becoming more short of breath and his oxygen saturations are decreasing to 70% on high-flow oxygen. When you arrive he is gasping for breath and appears very unwell. On examination he is tachypnoeic, using accessory muscles of respiration, and has crackles bilaterally to above the mid-zones. His heart rate is over 100 per minute and is irregular with a raised JVP. You administer morphine and intravenous diuretic, which leads to a slight improvement. Which ONE of the following should be considered next?**

- A Digoxin
- B Dobutamine
- C GTN infusion
- D Adrenaline
- E CPAP

questions

K104 **A patient involved in a road traffic accident is brought in with severe respiratory distress to the Emergency Department. On examination the trachea is deviated to the right with a hyper-resonant percussion note on the left. What is the next most appropriate step?**

○ A 100% inspired oxygen until senior help arrives

○ B Chest drain insertion

○ C Urgent chest X-ray

○ D Needle aspiration in 5th intercostal space, mid-axillary line

○ E Needle aspiration in 2nd intercostal space, mid-clavicular line

K105 **In which ONE of the following conditions is the water deprivation test most commonly used?**

○ A SIADH

○ B Hyponatraemic hypovolaemia

○ C ACTH-dependent Cushing's disease

○ D Renal tubular acidosis

○ E Diabetes insipidus

K106 **Which ONE of the following best indicates immunity in those receiving the hepatitis B vaccine?**

○ A Hepatitis B surface antigen

○ B Hepatitis B e antigen

○ C Anti-HBs antibody

○ D Anti-HBc antibody

○ E Anti-HBe antibody

K107 **An 18-year-old basketball player presents to the Emergency Department with shortness of breath and pleuritic chest pain. A chest X-ray shows a 1.5-cm rim of air between the pleurae with absent lung markings at the apex. There is no significant respiratory distress and he is much more comfortable after pain relief. Which ONE of the following should be the next step in his management?**

    A Discharge

    B Chest drain

    C Aspiration

    D Admit to ensure complete resolution

    E Pleurodesis

K108 **A 32-year-old insurance saleswoman presents to the Emergency Department after being found by her husband with an empty bottle of tablets and a half-finished bottle of vodka. The husband says that she has seen the GP regularly because of depression but does not know what the tablets were for. On examination her pupils are dilated but responsive to light, her mucous membranes and tongue appear dry and she is in sinus tachycardia. Which ONE of the following is most useful initially to assess the severity of the overdose?**

    A Drug levels

    B Liver function tests

    C Activated charcoal

    D ECG

    E INR

ANSWERS ON PAGE 240

K109 **A 50-year-old musician presents with significant haemoptysis that has been getting progressively worse over the past few weeks. This has been accompanied by a troublesome cough, wheezing and chest pain. He also says that he suffers from recurrent episodes of nosebleeds and haematuria. Chest X-ray shows multiple masses in both lung fields and urine dipstick is positive for blood and protein. What is the most likely diagnosis?**

○ A Systemic lupus erythematosus
○ B Aspergillosis
○ C Widespread metastatic disease
○ D Vasculitis
○ E Warfarin overdose

K110 **A 24-year-old university student presents to his GP with worsening rhinorrhoea and cough, and reports that his sense of taste has deteriorated and that he cannot smell things easily. He has come to the practice today because his girlfriend has told him that he has been snoring more over the past few weeks and because he is feeling more tired. He is otherwise well, apart from seasonal asthma which is controlled well with salbutamol. Which ONE of the following is the most appropriate step in the management of this patient?**

○ A Reassure and discharge
○ B Arrange for overnight oximetry and sleep studies
○ C Referral to a respiratory physician
○ D Surgical referral
○ E Optimise his asthma medications, starting with the introduction of a steroid inhaler

ANSWERS ON PAGE 241

K111 A 35-year-old software engineer presents to you with a long history of diarrhoea, which on further questioning you learn to be steatorrhoea. This has been accompanied by weight loss and fever, although the first symptom was joint pains. On examination he has widespread peripheral lymphadenopathy with ophthalmoplegia and nystagmus. Which ONE of the following would be diagnostic for the above condition?

○ A Small-bowel biopsy

○ B MRI head

○ C Barium follow-through

○ D CT abdomen

○ E Bone marrow biopsy

K112 A patient with early gastric cancer is admitted for a gastrectomy under the care of your consultant. Which ONE of the following is the most suitable for postoperative pain relief?

○ A Regular long-acting oral morphine with as-required Oramorph

○ B Epidural anaesthesia

○ C Spinal anaesthesia

○ D Intercostal nerve block

○ E Patient-controlled analgesia

K113 **A patient is started on steroids for an exacerbation of COPD; he has been admitted on numerous occasions throughout the past year and has had numerous courses of steroids and is concerned about the side-effects he has read about on the internet. Which ONE of the following is *not* a side-effect of steroid use?**

○ A Hyperkalaemia

○ B Acne

○ C Euphoria

○ D Amenorrhoea

○ E Dyspepsia

K114 **You are an F2 in a general practice and are seeing a patient with terminal cancer who requires pain relief. Which ONE of the following is *not* required on a controlled drug prescription?**

○ A Address of general practice

○ B Number of tablets in words

○ C Dosage in words

○ D Date written by hand

○ E 'Dental treatment only' written if issued by a dentist

ANSWERS ON PAGE 242

K115 **A 25-year-old model comes to see you in general practice because of a strange distribution of hair loss, which is causing him problems with work. On examination he has two well-defined areas of hair loss on the scalp with normal hair growth on the face and body. On inspection of the hair near the lesion, the hair strands seem to become thinner proximally. Examination of the hands reveals pitting of the nails. Which ONE of the following is most likely in this patient?**

○ A Self-inflicted hair loss

○ B Alopecia areata

○ C Psoriasis

○ D Scalp ringworm

○ E Lichen planus

K116 **You are the F2 in the Surgical Outpatient Clinic and have been asked to see Mr Smith by the consultant. Mr Smith is a 58-year-old gentleman who presents with trouble defecating and although he is still passes his motions normally, over the past month he has noticed the uncomfortable feeling of still wanting to defecate after passing his motions. During the past 2 weeks he has noticed that he has been passing mucus but denies any blood or change in colour. What is the next most appropriate step?**

○ A Colonoscopy

○ B Barium enema

○ C Faecal occult blood testing

○ D Sigmoidoscopy

○ E CT abdomen

K117 A 67-year-old patient admitted with acute heart failure develops tinnitus and difficulty hearing. Which ONE of the following is most likely to have led to this complication?

○ A Digoxin
○ B Ramipril
○ C Gentamicin
○ D Furosemide
○ E Spironolactone

K118 Which ONE of the following is a good prognostic variable in patients with schizophrenia?

○ A Early age of onset
○ B Acute onset
○ C Negative symptoms
○ D Male sex
○ E Poor adjustment

K119 A patient is having their JVP monitored: you note that the JVP is raised with a normal waveform. Which ONE of the following is most likely to lead to this picture?

○ A Iatrogenic
○ B Superior vena cava obstruction
○ C Pulmonary stenosis
○ D Complete heart block
○ E Constrictive pericarditis

ANSWERS ON PAGES 243–244

K120 **Which ONE of the following risk factors is responsible for the greatest number of patients with atrial fibrillation?**

○ A Hypertension

○ B Diabetes mellitus

○ C Ischaemic heart disease

○ D Thyrotoxicosis

○ E Normal ageing

K121 **You are in the Endoscopy Suite assisting the registrar with a difficult colonoscopy. While engrossed in the procedure the pulse oximeter reading drops to 80% and remains that way for 2 minutes despite adjusting the probe. Which ONE of the following medications should be on standby?**

○ A Midazolam

○ B Flumazenil

○ C Glucagon

○ D Calcium gluconate

○ E Doxapram

K122 **A 12-year-old boy presents with haematuria with a mild fever. Blood is present throughout the stream and he denies any dysuria or burning. Urine dipstick showed evidence of blood and protein. On questioning the mother you learn that he had a pharyngitis-like illness 2 weeks previously. Which ONE of the following diagnoses is most likely in this patient?**

○ A Berger's disease

○ B Buerger's disease

○ C Post-streptococcal glomerulonephritis

○ D Renal stones

○ E Early Henoch–Schönlein purpura

ANSWERS ON PAGES 244–245

questions

K123 **A patient is brought into the Emergency Department unwell and pyrexial at 38.5 °C. You are unable to gain a detailed history and initial examination is unremarkable. You take a brief history and perform blood tests which show raised inflammatory markers with a pancytopenia:**

Haemoglobin	9 g/dl
Lymphocyte count	$0.9 \times 10^9/l$
Neutrophil count	$0.5 \times 10^9/l$

Which ONE of the following should be undertaken?

○ A Benzylpenicillin and flucloxacillin intravenously

○ B Paracetamol and intravenous fluids until culture results are available

○ C Metronidazole and cefuroxime intravenously

○ D Tazocin and gentamicin intravenously

○ E Aciclovir intravenously

K124 **Which ONE of the following statements is true with regard to cranial nerves?**

○ A A lesion of the twelfth cranial nerve leads to the deviation of the tongue away from the side of the lesion

○ B The glossopharyngeal nerve is responsible for the efferent pathway of the gag reflex

○ C A peripheral lesion of the trigeminal nerve leads to deviation of the jaw towards the side of the lesion

○ D Gradenigo syndrome leads to an ipsilateral occulomotor nerve lesion

○ E The seventh cranial nerve carries sympathetic nerve fibres

K125 A 49-year-old lady is brought into the Emergency Department because of difficulty breathing. On examination she has decreased movement of the right side of her chest with absent breath sounds and dullness to percussion. A therapeutic and diagnostic procedure is undertaken which is then analysed according to Light's criteria. Which ONE of the following is *not* in the same class as the others when the results of the above procedure are analysed?

○ A Pneumonia
○ B Cirrhosis
○ C Pancreatitis
○ D SLE
○ E Mesothelioma

K126 A patient is allergic to penicillin, developing swelling of the lips when taken. Which ONE of the following antibiotics is safest to use?

○ A Augmentin
○ B Cefuroxime
○ C Ceftriaxone
○ D Ciprofloxacin
○ E Tazocin

K127 Which ONE of the following does *not* occur with osteoarthritis?

○ A Joint enubriation
○ B Osteophyte formation
○ C Ankylosis
○ D Joint space narrowing
○ E Subchondral cysts

K128 **A 30-year-old college student undergoes a flexible sigmoidoscopy for diarrhoea that has been occurring on and off for the past few years. She reports bloating and abdominal cramps but no other symptoms. The flexible sigmoidoscopy shows melanosis coli. Which ONE of the following is the most likely diagnosis?**

A Hyperthyroidism

B Laxative abuse

C Coeliac disease

D Microscopic colitis

E Malignancy

K129 **A 32-year-old patient who is 20 weeks pregnant presents with excessive sweating, tremor, weight loss and feeling hot all the time. On examination she has lid lag and exophthalmos. Which ONE of the following is the most suitable treatment option?**

A Radioactive iodine

B Thyroidectomy

C Carbimazole

D Propranolol

E Propylthiouracil

ANSWERS ON PAGE 247

K130 You are an F2 on a care-of-the-elderly ward in a busy district general hospital. A patient, Mr Brown, is under your care and was admitted because of acute-onset confusion. An abbreviated mental test score undertaken in the Emergency Department was 6/10 and you are asked to undertake a mini mental state examination. Which ONE of the following is part of the MMSE?

○ A Repeat the phrase 'West Registry Street'
○ B Ask the patient which year World War I started
○ C Identify and name two objects
○ D Ask the patient to draw two interlocking quadrangles
○ E Repeat the phrase 'No ifs, ors and buts'

K131 You are an F1 in gastroenterology and are admitting a patient with jaundice. Which ONE of the following statements with regard to this sign is true?

○ A Jaundice is usually clinically detectable with bilirubin concentrations greater than 80 µmol/l
○ B Gilbert syndrome and Crigler–Najjar syndrome lead to jaundice through defects in the same enzyme
○ C An ALT:AST ratio of 2 or more heavily suggests alcohol abuse
○ D Anti-mitochondrial antibodies are specific to primary biliary cirrhosis
○ E Bilirubin is converted to urobilinogen by the liver

questions

K132 **A patient is sent to hospital by her general practitioner because of pneumonia. Which ONE of the following features is an indicator of severe pneumonia?**

○ A Confusion

○ B Creatinine of 150 µmol/l

○ C Respiratory rate of < 10/minute

○ D Bradycardia < 70/minute

○ E Age > 60

K133 **An elderly gentleman is seen by a hospital consultant for general malaise and weakness. He reports early-morning stiffness and muscle ache, worse in his upper limbs compared with his lower limbs. He also states that he has lost weight and is becoming increasingly more depressed. The consultant makes the correct diagnosis and institutes the appropriate therapy. Which ONE of the following statements is true?**

○ A The disease responds to prednisolone treatment

○ B Morning stiffness is not in keeping with the other symptoms

○ C There is a male preponderance

○ D Normal inflammatory markers would be seen

○ E The disease incidence peaks at age 45

ANSWERS ON PAGES 249–250

K134 **A 28-year-old woman is referred to the Neurology Clinic because of recurrent headaches associated with sweating and anxiety. She is noted to be tachycardic and markedly hypertensive by the neurologist despite being started on multiple antihypertensive medications by her general practitioner. Which ONE of the following is most useful in this patient to diagnose the underlying condition?**

A CT head

B Psychiatric referral

C ECG

D Blood test

E Urine test

K135 **A 52-year-old musician has been seen in clinic for a number of years because of worsening renal failure. Which ONE of the following is *least* likely to be used in the management of this patient?**

A Serial urea and creatinine measurements

B Oral phosphate binders

C Oral erythropoietin

D Regular weight measurements

E HMG-CoA reductase inhibitor

ANSWERS ON PAGE 250

115

K136 With regard to COPD, which ONE of the following statements is true?

A   Tiotropium is a long-acting inhaled theophylline preparation

B   Inhaled corticosteroids should be started in patients to decrease exacerbations when the FEV_1 is less than 75% of predicted

C   Night-time waking with breathlessness is a common finding in COPD patients

D   Patients who still remain breathless after maximal medical therapy should be considered for surgery

E FEV_1 and FEV_1/FVC would be expected to return to normal in patients with COPD treated with maximal medical therapy

K137 Which ONE of the following is most suggestive of chronic renal failure as opposed to acute renal failure?

A   Anaemia

B   Gastritis

C   Creatinine > 1000 µmol/l

D   Hyperkalaemia

E   Small kidneys

K138 **Which ONE of the following statements about Parkinson's disease is true?**

○ A There is a higher incidence in females

○ B There is increased amplitude of tremor in sleep and decreased amplitude on mental exertion

○ C Levodopa is combined routinely with COMT inhibitors to increase availability of levodopa to the brain

○ D The presence of dementia at diagnosis is highly suggestive

○ E Rigidity is worsened with voluntary movement of the contralateral limb

K139 **You are reviewing patients in the Hepatology Clinic along with your consultant. Which ONE of the following is true?**

○ A The leading cause of cirrhosis worldwide is alcohol

○ B In Budd–Chiari syndrome there is obstruction of the portal vein

○ C Schistosomiasis can lead to pre-hepatic portal hypertension

○ D Patients with primary biliary cirrhosis typically have raised serum cholesterol levels

○ E Non-alcoholic steatohepatitis is a benign condition

K140 **A 55-year-old patient recently attended his general practitioner for his annual check-up and was found to have a normal examination, but routine blood tests revealed hypercholesterolaemia. Which ONE of the following statements is true?**

○ A Fibrates are agonists of the PPAR-α receptor and raise HDL cholesterol levels

○ B Familial hypercholesterolaemia is the commonest cause of elevated cholesterol levels in the population

○ C Ezetimibe inhibits hepatic uptake of cholesterol by interfering with LDL receptor expression

○ D Familial hypercholesterolaemia is autosomal recessive in its inheritance

○ E The incidence of hypercholesterolaemia in relation to age has a normal distribution

K141 **An 82-year-old lady with a past medical history of transient ischaemic attacks comes to see you in clinic with increasing tiredness. She is in rate-controlled atrial fibrillation and her medications include aspirin, omeprazole and digoxin. You order routine blood tests which reveal a haemoglobin of 8.9 g/dl and an MCV of 73 fl. Which ONE of the following is the correct option for her further management?**

○ A Start ferrous sulphate 200 mg three times a day

○ B Measure serum ferritin

○ C Measure serum iron and total iron-binding capacity

○ D Colonoscopy and endoscopy

○ E Repeat blood test in 1 month

K142 A 64-year-old gentleman presents with weight gain, lethargy and constipation. He is also more intolerant of the cold and wears a number of layers, even indoors. He is being treated with a number of medications for poorly controlled atrial fibrillation. His past medical history is one of asthma, for which he takes salbutamol inhalers as required and hypercholesterolaemia, for which he is on a statin. Which ONE of the following medications is most likely to account for the above symptoms?

○ A Simvastatin

○ B Amiodarone

○ C Digoxin

○ D Beta-blockers

○ E Verapamil

K143 A 54-year-old gentleman presents to the Emergency Department with increasing shortness of breath and basal crepitations. He is treated for heart failure with a number of medications and an echocardiogram is arranged to assess left ventricular function. While awaiting this investigation he develops swelling and severe pain in his right wrist associated with swelling and mild erythema of the overlying skin. On examination he is apyrexial and the heart failure remains under good control. Blood tests show no evidence of an infection. Which ONE of the following is most useful in this patient?

○ A Allopurinol

○ B Ibuprofen

○ C Aspirin

○ D Colchicine

○ E Naproxen

K144 **A 25-year-old pizza delivery motorcyclist is involved in a road traffic accident and suffers significant head trauma. You are the F2 in the Emergency Department and are worried about rising intracranial pressure. Which ONE of the following is *not* in keeping with this diagnosis?**

○ A Sixth cranial nerve lesion
○ B Confusion and aggression
○ C Bradycardia
○ D Hypotension
○ E Cheynes–Stokes respiration

K145 **You are an F2 in the Emergency Department of a busy district general hospital and a patient who has taken an overdose is brought in by ambulance. You are considering administering activated charcoal for the overdose. Which ONE of the following overdoses can be treated with activated charcoal?**

○ A Iron
○ B Methanol
○ C Lithium
○ D Aminophylline
○ E Ethylene glycol

ANSWERS ON PAGES 253–254

K146 A 27-year-old architect student presents with significant haemoptysis and bloodstained urine. This is accompanied by arthralgia and a mild pyrexia. A chest X-ray performed shows lower-lobe infiltration and renal function shows marked deterioration. Which ONE of the following tests is the most useful in this patient?

○ A Anti-rheumatoid factor antibodies
○ B Anti-Ro antibodies
○ C Anti-glomerular basement membrane antibodies
○ D Anti-double-stranded DNA antibodies
○ E Serum ACE

K147 A 15-year-old schoolgirl presents with central abdominal pain that localises to the right lower quadrant. This is accompanied by decreased appetite, a pyrexia of 37.6 °C and nausea. Which ONE of the following statements is true with regard to this condition?

○ A Mortality is highest for patients aged between 10 and 20 years
○ B Pain on palpation of the right iliac fossa but not on the left iliac fossa is known as Rovsig's sign
○ C Diabetic ketoacidosis is an important differential diagnosis
○ D Lymphocytosis is present in between 80% and 90% of patients
○ E A positive urine test for βhCG rules out the above condition

K148 **A 24-year-old attends the Emergency Department with a tender erythematous rash on his shins accompanied by arthralgia and fevers. He is originally from Turkey and is studying at university in the UK. He had visited his GP a few days earlier, who felt that this was a viral infection. On examination there are multiple ulcers within the mouth and on the scrotum and there is a raised erythematous papule in the right antecubital fossa, which was the site of a blood test from 2 days ago. Which ONE of the following is the most likely disease?**

- A AIDS-related phenomenon
- B Tuberculosis
- C Kawasaki disease
- D Behçet's disease
- E Herpes simplex

K149 **You are an F1 in general internal medicine and are reviewing a 76-year-old lady who was brought into the Emergency Department confused and disorientated. Routine blood tests show that she has a sodium of 125 mmol/l. Which ONE of the following investigations is *least* useful?**

- A Plasma lipids and glucose
- B Thyroid functions tests
- C Dexamethasone suppression test
- D Urine sodium
- E Urine osmolality

K150 A 36-year-old lady is brought in by ambulance after being taken unwell in a local shopping centre. On examination she is drowsy, confused and sweating profusely, with a pyrexia of 38.5 °C. She is tachypnoeic with a respiratory rate of 30/minute and is tachycardic with a rate of 120/minute and in atrial fibrillation. She has been seen previously in the thyroid clinic. Which ONE of the following should *not* be given to this patient initially?

○ A Lugol's iodine
○ B Propylthiouracil
○ C Hydrocortisone
○ D Propanolol
○ E 10% glucose

K151 A patient presents to the Respiratory Department after undergoing lung function tests ordered by his general practitioner. Of note, the FEV_1 was 1.75 litres and the FVC was 2 litres. Which diagnosis is *least* likely in the above patient?

○ A Pneumoconiosis
○ B Sarcoidosis
○ C Cystic fibrosis
○ D Obesity
○ E Myasthenia gravis

K152 You are an F2 on call in a busy district general hospital for general surgery and get bleeped at 10pm to see a 45-year-old chef who recently underwent a laparotomy for resection of diseased small bowel secondary to Crohn's disease. The nurses state that he is complaining of not being able to move his legs and his observations are: temperature 37.0 °C, heart rate 50/minute, BP 105/60 mmHg, respiratory rate 15/minute and saturation on room air 97%. He is receiving bupivacaine analgesia through an epidural which is working well. When you go to see him he appears totally pain-free and examination of his legs reveals that they are completely paralysed. Which ONE of the following is true?

- A   The on-call surgical registrar should be informed
- B   The patient is at risk of metabolic alkalosis
- C   Sitting the patient upright is contraindicated
- D   The epidural should be slowed but kept running
- E   Naloxone would be helpful

K153 A 20-year-old architect student is brought to see you by his family because they are concerned about his behaviour. He has recently lost his temper with a number of friends, colleagues and family members and has started to become forgetful. You note that he has a resting tremor and has uncontrolled writhing movements of his left hand. Blood tests show deranged liver function tests. Which ONE of the following is the most important initial investigation?

- A   EEG
- B   Psychiatric review for alcohol abuse
- C   Blood test
- D   Urine test
- E   Reassurance

ANSWERS ON PAGE 256

K154 **A 22-year-old semi-professional football player comes to see you because of pain and discharge near his anus. He tells you that it is extremely tender and sore and discharging pus. Apart from this he has no other complaints and his systems review is unremarkable. Abdominal examination shows no abnormalities but examination of the area around his anus shows a discharging sinus in the intergluteal cleft 5 cm from the anus, with an area of overlying erythema, most likely due to an abscess. Which ONE of the following statements is true?**

○ A There is a racial difference, with this condition being more common in Africans and Asians

○ B Incision and drainage of the abscess is recommended in this patient

○ C Women are usually affected later than men

○ D Obesity is a protective factor in developing this condition

○ E Meticulous shaving and hygiene has no role in the control of this disease

K155 **What is the commonest cause of death in patients with Parkinson's disease?**

○ A Accidental injury

○ B Myocardial infarction

○ C Bronchopneumonia

○ D Stroke

○ E Dementia

ANSWERS ON PAGES 256–257

K156 A 45-year-old lady presents to the general practitioner complaining of itching under her breasts. Her height is 1.75 m and her weight is 150 kg; examination of the breasts reveals no obvious asymmetry and no masses are palpable in the breasts or in the axilla. On examination of the underside of her breasts there was an erythematous and warm rash with significant excoriation marks. A few vesicles could be seen. Which ONE of the following is most important with regard to her longer-term health?

- A Microbiology sample for culture, sensitivity and microscopy
- B Steroid cream
- C Blood glucose measurement
- D Aqueous cream
- E Thyroid function tests

K157 You are the F1 in the Emergency Department and are asked to see a patient who was referred by their GP following an overdose. On speaking to the 25-year-old patient you learn that she recently failed her final university exams and took an unspecified number of aspirin tablets from her grandmother's cupboard. Which ONE of the following statements with regard to aspirin overdose is true?

- A A respiratory alkalosis would be in keeping with this overdose
- B Aspirin overdose is relatively asymptomatic in the first 24 hours
- C Paracetamol levels are not required
- D Plasma concentrations are not helpful in assessing the severity of poisoning
- E Chronic but not acute renal failure is a complication of aspirin overdose

ANSWERS ON PAGE 257

K158 A 30-year-old cyclist was enjoying a brisk ride through central London when he was involved in a road traffic accident. He is brought into the Emergency Department complaining of severe chest pain secondary to the collision. A chest X-ray shows no fractures but does reveal an enlarged heart border. An echocardiogram is diagnostic. Which ONE of the following would *not* be in keeping with the diagnosis?

○ A Muffled heart sounds

○ B Significant drop in jugular venous pressure on inspiration

○ C Falling blood pressure

○ D Pulsus paradoxus

○ E Electrical alternans on ECG

K159 A long-standing diabetic is brought into the Emergency Department by his son, who says that is father is very unwell. He is pyrexial, delirious and appears jaundiced. He is well known to the Diabetic Foot Clinic, where he is seen regularly for his neuropathic foot ulcers. His son reports that his father suffered a fall yesterday and sustained considerable bruising and cuts to his legs. On removing the bandages the left lower leg is very oedematous and erythematous and crepitations can be heard on palpation. Which ONE of the following is responsible?

○ A MRSA

○ B Tetanus

○ C *Clostridium botulinum*

○ D *Enterococcus faecalis*

○ E *Clostridium perfringens*

K160 **A 4-year-old boy complains of itching, especially at night, and is brought to see you in general practice by his father. He has marked excoriation marks over his face with an underlying macular rash and a rash on the flexor surfaces of both his wrists and around his umbilicus. There are also excoriations in the web spaces of the hands, but the father reports that none of the other family members have been affected. He reports that when he was a baby the child had severe napkin dermatitis. Which ONE of the following is the most likely diagnosis?**

○ A Eczema

○ B Psoriasis

○ C Scabies

○ D Bed bugs

○ E Chickenpox

K161 **A patient was admitted with an acute exacerbation of severe COPD that required HDU admission. He made a gradual recovery and was transferred to the ward, where he was given maximal medical therapy. He was thought to be a candidate for long-term oxygen therapy (LTOT). Which ONE of the following is true with regard to LTOT?**

○ A Patients should be advised to keep oxygen on for more than 5 hours every day

○ B Mortality is decreased by 10% compared with those not receiving treatment

○ C Two arterial blood gas readings, one on admission and one 3 weeks later are needed to assess suitability for LTOT

○ D Patients should have a PaO_2 less than 7.3 kPa to be suitable for LTOT

○ E Polycythaemia increases the PaO_2 threshold for patients to receive LTOT

ANSWERS ON PAGE 258

K162 **Which ONE of the following suggests a diagnosis other than migraine?**

○ A Paraesthesia
○ B Scalp tenderness
○ C Ataxia
○ D Coincides with periods
○ E Allodynia

K163 **A 75-year-old lady in brought into the Emergency Department because of pain in her back, which is tender to palpation. Her blood results show a degree of inflammation, although no focus of infection can be identified. Her urea and creatinine are both raised, with a urea of 15 mmol/l and a creatinine of 236 μmol/l while her sodium is 132 mmol/l, potassium 3.3 mmol/l and corrected calcium 2.98 mmol/l. Which ONE of the following is most useful is establishing the underlying diagnosis?**

○ A Serum free light chains
○ B Serum vitamin D concentration
○ C Serum parathyroid concentration
○ D Renal ultrasound
○ E Chest X-ray

K164 **Which ONE of the following is *not* a sinister feature when assessing the likelihood of spinal cord compression in someone complaining of sudden-onset back pain?**

- ○ A Age of 40
- ○ B Gait disturbance
- ○ C Pyrexia of unknown origin
- ○ D Weight loss
- ○ E Prostate cancer

K165 **You are an F2 in the Emergency Department 30 minutes from a tertiary referral centre. An ambulance is en route with a stable patient with known ST-elevation myocardial infarction. Which ONE of the following is the best option?**

- ○ A The ambulance should take the patient to the tertiary referral centre for primary percutaneous coronary intervention
- ○ B The patient should be brought to the Emergency Department for thrombolysis
- ○ C The patient should be brought to the Emergency Department for thrombolysis and then transferred to the tertiary centre for percutaneous coronary intervention
- ○ D As the patient is stable he can be taken to the tertiary referral centre for thrombolysis and primary percutaneous coronary intervention
- ○ E The paramedics should administer thrombolytics with subsequent follow-up at the tertiary referral centre

ANSWERS ON PAGES 259–260

K166 **A patient is referred to the Emergency Department by their general practitioner for severe ulcerative colitis. Which ONE of the following is *not* a marker of severity?**

○ A Tachycardia

○ B Stool consistency

○ C Stool frequency

○ D Fever > 37.5 °C

○ E Albumin < 30 g/dl

K167 **Which ONE of the following is true with regard to pernicious anaemia?**

○ A The presence of thyroid autoantibodies implies an alternative diagnosis

○ B Patients are at decreased risk of gastric cancer

○ C It is associated with blood group A

○ D Intrinsic factor antibodies are present in 90% of patients

○ E Parietal cell antibodies are diagnostic

K168 A 58-year-old hospital porter presents to you with muscle weakness and pain that has been causing him great difficulty. On examination the cardiovascular, respiratory and abdominal examinations are unremarkable but weakness is noted on neurological examination, with preservation of the reflexes. While examining the hands you note roughened red papules over the extensor surfaces of the phalanges. Blood tests show normal thyroid function and liver function and no evidence of anaemia. Rheumatoid factor is negative but creatine kinase is significantly raised. Which ONE of the following is most likely?

   A Side-effect from statins

   B Rheumatoid arthritis

   C Psoriatic arthropathy

   D Dermatomyositis

   E SLE

K169 You are reviewing a 35-year-old gentleman in the Gastroenterology Clinic who has been referred by his general practitioner with suspected inflammatory bowel disease. You suspect Crohn's disease and your consultant asks you which site is most commonly affected in Crohn's disease?

   A Ileocaecal valve

   B Rectum

   C Sigmoid colon

   D Small bowel

   E Oesophagus

ANSWERS ON PAGE 261

K170 A 35-year-old lady presents to her general practitioner with recurrent attacks of vertigo which she describes as quite disabling. This is accompanied by a loud ringing sensation in her ears and deafness. Which ONE of the following is most likely in this patient?

- A Vestibular neuronitis
- B Ménière's disease
- C Middle ear infection
- D Viral labrynthitis
- E Eight cranial nerve palsy

K171 An 80-year-old widower presents to the Emergency Department after a mechanical fall at a local store. Orthopaedic examination is unremarkable but he is very thin and restless, suffers from halitosis and gingivitis and perifollicular haemorrhages can be seen. What is the likely diagnosis?

- A Vitamin K deficiency
- B Vitamin C deficiency
- C Lead poisoning
- D Hypothyroidism
- E Pellagra

K172 Which ONE of the following occurs in aortic regurgitation?

○ A Hyperdynamic apex

○ B Diastolic murmur heard best while the patient is leaning forwards on inspiration

○ C De Mullet's sign

○ D Narrow pulse pressure

○ E Graham Steell murmur

K173 A 76-year-old lady comes to see her GP with her daughter, who reports that her mother has been feeling down for the past 3 months and also getting easily upset, forgetful and confused. She reports that her mother has had diarrhoea for a number of weeks. On examination you note a rash on her hands and in a 'V' distribution on her chest. Which ONE of the following is the most likely diagnosis?

○ A Scurvy

○ B Coeliac disease

○ C Depression

○ D Pellagra

○ E Pseudo-dementia

K174 Which ONE of the following features is more in keeping with myasthenia gravis than with a diagnosis of Eaton–Lambert syndrome?

○ A Associated lung cancer

○ B Proximal limb and trunk weakness

○ C Autonomic involvement

○ D Repeated muscle contraction leading to fatigue

○ E Hyporeflexia

134

ANSWERS ON PAGE 262

K175 **Which ONE of the following is *not* part of the metabolic syndrome?**

O   A   Hypertension
O   B   Hypercholesterolaemia
O   C   Raised LDL cholesterol
O   D   Abdominal obesity
O   E   Impaired fasting glucose

K176 **A 37-year-old housewife presents with facial pain worse on leaning forwards which is accompanied by a feeling of pressure over the right side of her face. Her husband comments that she has developed bad breath over the past few weeks and she complains of altered taste of food. Which ONE of the following statements is true with regard to this condition?**

O   A   The frontal sinuses are most commonly affected
O   B   In chronic cases radiographs are as useful as CT scans of the affected region
O   C   Exacerbation when leaning forwards should alert you to an alternative diagnosis
O   D   Viral upper respiratory tract infections are the most common predisposing factor in the development of the condition
O   E   *Moraxella catarrhalis* is the commonest bacterial pathogen involved in children

questions

K177 Occlusion of the middle cerebral artery leads to all of the following EXCEPT?

○ A Contralateral hemiplegia, in the upper limb more than the lower

○ B Eyes deviate away from the lesion

○ C Global aphasia

○ D Homonymous hemianopia

○ E Drowsiness and stupor

K178 With regard to hypertrophic obstructive cardiomyopathy which ONE of the statements below is *false*?

○ A Can be inherited in an autosomal dominant fashion

○ B Worse prognosis if aged over 20 years at presentation

○ C Presents with symptoms of aortic stenosis

○ D Presents with sudden death

○ E ECG can demonstrate pathological Q waves

ANSWERS ON PAGE 263

K179 **You are a doctor who decides to undertake a period of clinical training in rural India. A small boy aged approximately 12 years old is brought to you with a range of symptoms including fever, joint pains and malaise. On examination he has multiple swollen, tender and painful joints in a wide distribution but no visible rash. Auscultation reveals a diastolic murmur, with vesicular breath sounds in both lung fields. Which ONE of the following statements regarding this condition is true?**

○ A It is associated with group B β-haemolytic *Streptococcus*

○ B The vesicular breath sounds are classically associated with the disease

○ C Involvement of the central nervous system is more common in females

○ D An ECG has no role in the diagnosis of the condition

○ E Aspirin is contraindicated in the condition

K180 **Which ONE of the following is *least* useful in determining the cause of cirrhosis?**

○ A Serum autoantibodies

○ B Iron studies

○ C Copper studies

○ D α1-Antitrypsin

○ E Prothrombin time

questions

K181 **Which ONE of the following statements is true with regard to infliximab?**

○ A Patients should be screened for past exposure to tuberculosis

○ B It works by stopping tumour necrosis factor beta exerting its effects

○ C Methotrexate should be stopped as it counteracts the effect of infliximab

○ D Infliximab is usually started in general practice, with hospital follow-up

○ E It is used solely in rheumatology, dermatology and oncology

K182 **You are an F2 in cardiology and are reviewing a heart failure patient in clinic. Which ONE of the following has *not* been shown to improve survival in heart failure patients?**

○ A Ramipril
○ B Bisoprolol
○ C Spironolactone
○ D Bumetanide
○ E Nitrates with hydralazine

K183 **You are asked to review a patient with severe haemophilia A in the Emergency Department. Which ONE of the following is true with regard to haemophilia A?**

○ A In the majority of cases the patient's father would also be expected to suffer from the disease

○ B Levels of affected coagulation factor are less than 15% of normal in severely affected individuals

○ C Chromosome 8 is the location of the affected gene

○ D Desmopressin would be an effective treatment in the above patient

○ E The bleeding time is usually normal in patients with haemophilia A

K184 **An intravenous drug user is brought into the Emergency Department because of a swollen left leg which is warm and tender on examination. There is a 5-cm difference in circumference measurements between the two legs. The diagnosis is confirmed on imaging and you initiate therapy. There is some concern about compliance with medications and subsequent follow-up. Which ONE of the following is the most suitable treatment?**

○ A Warfarin

○ B High-dose aspirin

○ C Low-molecular-weight heparin

○ D Phenindione

○ E Unfractionated heparin

K185 A 22-year-old man presents with deterioration in his vision which has been getting worse over the past few hours. On examination, eye movements are painful and he reports colours that are not as bright and distinct as before. Fundoscopy reveals no abnormalities of the optic disc and macula. Which ONE of the following is the most likely diagnosis?

- A Somatisation
- B Migraine with aura
- C Optic neuritis
- D Uveitis
- E Scleritis

K186 A 30-year-old secretary presents to her general practitioner with lethargy and weakness. She states that she has developed worsening diplopia over the past few weeks and that her husband has commented on her eyelids becoming droopy. You note towards the end of the consultation that her speech has a nasal quality to it. Which ONE of the following is the most likely diagnosis?

- A Hypothyroidism
- B Pseudobulbar palsy
- C Myasthenia gravis
- D Myotonic dystrophy
- E Multiple sclerosis

ANSWERS ON PAGE 267

K187 **A 35-year-old patient presents to the Emergency Department with a range of symptoms, including visual blurring, tinnitus, dysarthria and perioral paraesthesia. The patient also complains of a throbbing headache and photophobia. Which ONE of the following is most likely?**

○ A Vertebral artery stroke
○ B Vertebral artery TIA
○ C Migraine
○ D Posterior inferior cerebellar artery thrombosis
○ E Cavernous sinus thrombosis

questions

K188 **A 50-year-old lady from West Africa presents to the Emergency Department with a range of symptoms, including weight loss and rashes, that have been ongoing for the past few years. She complains of lethargy and tiredness, with aches and pains in a range of her joints, and sore mouth ulcers. On examination she has a mild fever and is of thin build but cardiovascular and respiratory examinations are unremarkable. You arrange a number of blood tests, which are returned as showing:**

CRP	15 mg/l	Haemoglobin	8.4 g/dl
ESR	124 mm in 1st hour	WCC	4×10^9/l
Sodium	136 mmol/l	Platelets	132×10^9/l
Potassium	4.0 mmol/l		
Urea	10 mmol/l	Urinary blood	+ +
Creatinine	150 µmol/l	Urinary protein	+ + +
Calcium	2.25 mmol/l	Urinary glucose	+
TFTs	Normal	Urinary ketones	Negative
LFTs	Normal	Urinary nitrites	Negative

She is admitted for further observations and investigations and is found to have more than 5 g of protein in her 24-hour urine sample. Which ONE of the following is the most likely diagnosis?

A   Rheumatic fever

B   Systemic lupus erythematosus

C   HIV seroconversion

D   Chronic malaria

E   Nephrotic syndrome

ANSWER ON PAGE 267

K189 **A patient with known sickle cell disease presents to the Emergency Department with severe chest pain and difficulty breathing. Her oxygen saturations are 80% on high-flow oxygen and are deteriorating rapidly. You call the haematology team and the HDU. Which ONE of the following is most useful in this patient?**

O A Transfusion of O-negative blood

O B Exchange transfusion

O C Transfusion of FFP

O D Limited analgesia to prevent further respiratory depression

O E Hydroxyurea

K190 **Which ONE of the following statements is true?**

O A Bifascicular heart block manifests itself on ECG testing by the presence of right bundle branch block with left axis deviation

O B Delta waves are present on the ECG in hypothermic patients

O C Complete heart block with a broad-complex escape rhythm can be managed pharmacologically in most cases

O D Wenckebach AV block is a more unstable rhythm than Mobitz type II heart block

O E In first-degree heart block the delay occurs at the level of the sinoatrial node

K191 A 33-year-old woman presents to the Emergency Department with severe chest pain that she rates as 8/10 in severity. It is central in nature and slightly relieved when she sits upright. ECG shows widespread ST-segment elevation of more than 2 mm. She has a strong family history of ischaemic heart disease and death from heart attacks and strokes. Which ONE of the following is the best course of action?

○ A Thrombolysis

○ B Primary percutaneous angioplasty

○ C Echocardiogram

○ D High-dose steroids

○ E NSAIDs

K192 Which ONE of the following is *least* likely to occur as a complication of a myocardial infarction?

○ A Bradycardia

○ B Left ventricular aneurysm

○ C Ventricular septal defect

○ D Mitral stenosis

○ E Dressler syndrome

ANSWERS ON PAGE 269

K193 A recent study into the treatment of prostate cancer compared the use of a new drug X with conventional treatment. A total of 2000 subjects were randomised to receive either X with conventional treatment or conventional treatment alone (1000 in each arm). All patients were followed up for 10 years, with none being lost to follow-up. At the end of 10 years there were 600 patients alive in the conventional treatment alone arm whereas 800 patients were alive in the conventional treatment plus treatment X arm. What is the number needed to treat (NNT) with drug X to prevent one death?

○   A   5
○   B   10
○   C   15
○   D   20
○   E   50

K194 Which ONE of the following is the *least* important feature of screening?

○   A   Treatment should already exist for the condition being screened

○   B   The screening tool must identify an early stage of the disease

○   C   The screening tool must be highly sophisticated

○   D   Those at most risk should be identified and targeted

○   E   The disease being screened for should have a high healthcare burden

K195 A 62-year-old man who suffered from a myocardial infarction 2 months ago comes to see you in the clinic. He reports occasional episodes of feeling faint which occur at any time of day but which last only for a few seconds, however, he reports no chest pain. His legs have been getting progressively more swollen and he reports increasing orthopnoea despite maximal medical therapy and although he is comfortable at rest any small activity results in dyspnoea. His echocardiogram undertaken 1 month ago showed an ejection fraction of 20%–25% with akinesis of the inferior wall and marked dysynchrony. An ECG shows a left bundle branch block with a QRS duration of 145 ms. You arrange for a 24-hour tape, which shows short episodes of non-sustained ventricular tachycardia. Which ONE of the following is correct?

○ A The patient should have a biventricular pacemaker and implantable cardioverter defibrillator inserted

○ B The patient should have his beta-blockers stopped

○ C The patient should have a DDDR pacemaker inserted

○ D The patient should have an implantable cardioverter defibrillator inserted

○ E The patient should have electrophysiological studies performed, followed by radiofrequency ablation

ANSWER ON PAGE 270

K196 **A 36-year-old woman comes to see you in general practice because she is concerned about her health. In an effort to lose weight and become 'fit' she asks you about alcohol consumption. What is the maximum recommended amount of alcohol consumption for her per week?**

○ A 9 units

○ B 10 units

○ C 14 units

○ D 21 units

○ E 28 units

K197 **A 64-year-old lifelong smoker presents to the Emergency Department with shortness of breath. She is placed on controlled oxygen therapy and started on nebulised salbutamol and ipratropium bromide. On examination she is pyrexial, has a hyperinflated chest and has a few coarse crepitations at both lung bases, with limited air entry. Which ONE of the following options should also be considered?**

○ A Fluid restriction

○ B Physiotherapy

○ C Furosemide

○ D Maximum oxygen therapy

○ E Magnesium sulphate

K198 **A patient presents to the Emergency Department feeling generally unwell. Blood results show hyperkalaemia, hyperphosphataemia, hypocalcaemia, hypomagnesaemia and hyperuricaemia. He has recently been started on some treatment but you are not able to ascertain what this is for. Which ONE of the following is in keeping with the diagnosis?**

○ A Acute renal failure
○ B Superior vena cava obstruction
○ C Haemolytic uraemic syndrome
○ D Disseminated intravascular coagulation
○ E Tumour lysis syndrome

K199 **A 35-year-old gentleman has severe chest pain at a football match and collapses. He is rapidly brought into the Emergency Department, where he describes severe chest pain radiating to his back. On examination he is hypertensive, with weaker pulses on his left-hand side compared with the right. Which ONE of the following is the examination of choice in this patient?**

○ A Chest X-ray
○ B Carotid Doppler
○ C CT scan
○ D ECG
○ E Renal function tests

ANSWERS ON PAGE 271

K200 **During inflammation or infection the liver produces a number of acute phase proteins whose concentrations rise or fall as a response. Which ONE of the following is a negative acute phase protein?**

○ A CRP

○ B Ferritin

○ C α1-Antitrypsin

○ D Albumin

○ E Coagulation factors

K201 **A computer engineer presents to your general practice complaining of pain in the outer aspect of his arm. On examination, movement at the elbow is painful and tenderness can be demonstrated on palpation of the lateral border. The pain is worse when he picks up objects and relieved with rest and at night. Which ONE of the following is the patient most likely to be suffering from?**

○ A Golfer's elbow

○ B Tennis elbow

○ C Galeazzi fracture

○ D Repetitive strain injury

○ E Monteggia fracture

K202 **A patient attends the Emergency Department feeling generally unwell with abdominal pain, malaise, weakness and dizziness. On examination he looks tanned and is hypotensive, with a significant postural drop. Blood results are returned as: sodium 130 mmol/l, potassium 5.2 mmol/l and blood glucose 3.5 mmol/l. Which ONE of the following is the most common cause of these features?**

- A Autoimmune
- B Metastases
- C Tuberculosis
- D Genetic
- E Infective

K203 **A study was conducted that analyses the impact of television viewing on the BMI of children. It found that the relative risk of having a BMI > 30 if children watched more than 5 hours of television was 1.52 (95% confidence interval 1.28 to 2.10). Which ONE of the following statements is true?**

- A The more television children watch the higher their expected BMI
- B 52% of children who watch more than 5 hours of television will have a BMI of more than 30
- C The above results are based on a double-blinded randomised controlled trial
- D Advertising of high-fat foods should be limited based on the above study
- E The study is statistically and clinically significant

ANSWERS ON PAGE 272

K204 **You are working in the Hepatology Clinic and see a patient with known hepatitis B and hepatitis C. He is complaining of severe abdominal pain under the right costal margin, weight loss and increasing jaundice. An ultrasound scan is highly suggestive of the diagnosis. Which ONE of the following would be the most useful investigation?**

    A CEA

    B βhCG

    C αFP

    D CA-199

    E CA-125

K205 **You are an F2 in ophthalmology. Which ONE of the following statements is true?**

    A In a hypermetropic eye the point of maximal focus falls in front of the retina

    B Herpes simplex keratitis is effectively treated with topical steroid applications

    C Normal intraocular pressure is between 20 and 40 mmHg

    D Open angle glaucoma shows a wide racial preponderance, being 5–10 times more common in Afro-Caribbean patients compared with white patients

    E Xerophthalmia results from deficiency of vitamin E

K206 A 35-year-old patient undergoes a laparotomy due to a stab wound. The damaged bowel was resected, a primary anastamosis was made and the operation was deemed a success. The patient is given PCA pain relief by the anaesthetist and returned to the ward. On examination the next day the wound looks healthy and the drain that was inserted has collected 45 ml of bloodstained fluid. Nursing observations show a pyrexia of 37.6 °C and examination reveals decreased air entry at the bases. Abdominal examination reveals mild tenderness and bowel sounds are sparse. Which ONE of the following is most correct?

- A   The anastamosis is likely to be leaking
- B   The patient should have his antibiotics increased in view of the pyrexia
- C   The wound staples should be removed to aid healing
- D   Physiotherapy should be started early
- E   The patient is making a satisfactory recovery and no intervention is needed at this stage

K207 You are asked to review a chest X-ray of a patient admitted via the Emergency Department last night. You note tram-line shadowing and ring shadows. What is the most likely diagnosis?

- A   Sarcoidosis
- B   Pneumoconiosis
- C   Tuberculosis
- D   Bronchiectasis
- E   Consolidation

ANSWERS ON PAGE 273

K208 A patient attends his general practice because of pains in his upper limbs and neck which have been getting progressively worse. On examination you note a right Horner syndrome with wasting of the intrinsic muscles of the hands. His speech, visual fields and eye movements are normal, although sensation to pain and temperature is diminished in the upper limbs and trunk. Which ONE of the following is most likely?

○ A Pancoast's tumour

○ B Subacute combined degeneration of the spinal cord

○ C Syringobulbia

○ D Intrinsic cord lesion

○ E Tabes dorsalis

K209 A patient presents to the Inflammatory Bowel Disease Clinic with abdominal pain, jaundice and pruritis. On examination the patient is of slim build, hepatomegaly is present and an ill-defined solid mass is also found in the right upper quadrant of the abdomen. Liver function tests show raised bilirubin, alkaline phosphatase and γGT. An ERCP undertaken a number of years ago showed a beaded appearance of the bile ducts. What is the *underlying* diagnosis that accounts for the presentation and the mass in the right upper quadrant of the abdomen?

○ A Primary biliary cirrhosis

○ B Primary sclerosing cholangitis

○ C Autoimmune hepatitis

○ D Cholangiocarcinoma

○ E Hepatocellular carcinoma

K210 **A patient is brought to the Emergency Department from the local day-care hospital for older people because of sudden-onset vomiting, vertigo and unsteadiness. On examination there is demonstrable ataxia and nystagmus with loss of sensation to pinprick on the right side of the face but the left side of his trunk. Which ONE of the following is most likely?**

○ A Lateral medullary syndrome

○ B Gerstmann syndrome

○ C Labrynthitis

○ D Benign positional vertigo

○ E Subclavian steal syndrome

K211 **A patient presents to their general practitioner with slowly progressive hearing loss that is conductive in nature. In addition they complain of intermittent foul-smelling discharge, which is occasionally bloodstained. On examination you note that the nasolabial fold differs on his left and right sides. Otoscopy is diagnostic. Which ONE of the following is most likely?**

○ A Infiltrative *Pseudomonas* infection

○ B Otitis externa

○ C Chronic suppurative otitis media

○ D Cholesteatoma

○ E Squamous cell carcinoma of the external ear

K212 **A patient who is admitted late on Friday night is reviewed on the consultant ward round a few days later. The patient appears confused and agitated but is haemodynamically stable with no evidence of infection or dehydration. The patient denies being on any regular medication or taking any over-the-counter medications. Urgent blood tests show the following:**

Sodium	125 mmol/l
Potassium	2.5 mmol/l
Urea	3.6 mmol/l
Creatinine	70 µmol/l
Serum osmolality	255 mosmol/kg
Urine sodium	35 mmol/l
Urine osmolality	527 mosmol/kg

Which ONE of the following is most useful in the above patient?

A Desmopressin

B 0.45% saline

C Fluid restriction

D Venesection

E Chest X-ray

K213 **A 62-year-old man who was taking warfarin for a DVT sustained after an elective orthopaedic operation presents with black, tarry stools. On examination he is tachycardiac and has a postural blood pressure drop of 15 mmHg. The abdomen is soft and non-tender but there is melaena present on rectal examination. A blood test shows an INR of 7.2 and a haemoglobin level of 8.5 g/dl. Which ONE of the following is the most appropriate management?**

- A Prothrombin complex concentrates
- B Vitamin K 10 mg orally
- C Cryoprecipitate
- D Vitamin K 10 mg IV
- E Fresh frozen plasma

K214 **A patient presents to the Emergency Department feeling generally unwell with high fevers, weight loss and easy bruising. Routine blood tests are reported as markedly abnormal and a blood film reveals the presence of Auer rods. Which ONE of the following is the patient most likely to be suffering from?**

- A *Mycobacterium tuberculosis*
- B Chronic myeloid leukaemia
- C Acute myeloid leukaemia
- D Acute lymphocytic leukaemia
- E von Willebrand's disease

          ANSWERS ON PAGE 276

K215 A 40-year-old nurse who is originally from Zimbabwe is brought to the Emergency Department by his friends after acting strangely over the last few days (and more particularly over the past 24 hours). He has been shouting obscenities and has developed visual hallucinations. In addition, he has been confused and drowsy, has complained of headaches and has developed a pyrexia this evening. He was previously well, with no medical problems, though he did have a cold over the last week with a non-productive cough. Imaging has revealed no abnormalities on a chest X-ray but there are marked abnormalities in the left temporal region of the brain. Which ONE of the following is the most likely diagnosis?

O A *Mycobacterium tuberculosis* brain abscess

O B Rubella meningo-encephalitis

O C JC virus infection

O D HSV encephalitis

O E Temporal lobe epilepsy

K216 A 65-year-old man presents to his GP with a sensation of an irregular heart rhythm a few times a week. He says that he has felt his own pulse and found it to be irregular. You perform an ECG which confirms the diagnosis of atrial fibrillation at a rate of 55–70 beats per minute. His past medical history is significant for ischaemic heart disease, with two previous heart attacks and a coronary artery bypass operation 12 years ago. As result, he has congestive cardiac failure which is stable on medical therapy and has not required a hospital admission in 3 years. He has treated hypertension and diet-controlled diabetes but has never had a stroke and is otherwise fit and well and continues to work in the volunteer shop of the local hospital. Which ONE of the following would be the most appropriate therapy for primary stroke prevention?

- A Continue on aspirin 75 mg once daily
- B Increase aspirin to 300 mg once daily
- C Commence digoxin
- D Aspirin 75 mg once a day and dipyrimadole modified-release 200 mg twice a day
- E Initiate warfarin

ANSWERS

SECTION 1:
SCENARIO-BASED ANSWERS

Scenario 1

S1.1   E: Urine analysis

This patient presents with significant third-space fluid overload and although this could be cardiac in origin given her previous NSTEMI, her recent near-normal echocardiogram would not support this finding and repeating the echocardiogram would not be of any benefit.

The answer lies with the urine dipstick result, which shows proteinuria. This feature, the hypoalbuminaemia and the peripheral oedema comprise the classic features of nephrotic syndrome. Features supportive of nephrotic syndrome are the facial puffiness and hypercholesterolaemia. The most appropriate investigation is therefore a 24-hour urine collection or an albumin:creatinine ratio to quantify the extent of protein leak from the kidneys, followed by a renal biopsy.

Those of you who chose stem D (antibiotics), thinking this could represent a urinary tract infection because of the incontinence or cellulitis because of the erythematous legs should look carefully at all of the information. The incontinence is likely to be secondary to the diuretics rather than a UTI, while chronic leg swelling will result in erythema but does not necessarily imply cellulitis.

S1.2   C: There is increased susceptibility to infections

Patients with nephrotic syndrome are much more likely to develop infections which should be treated early and aggressively. Venous thromboembolism is also much more common in neprotic syndrome and prophylaxis with heparin is usual practice. ACE inhibitors limit protein leak and are generally continued and hypercholesterolaemia is a very commonly recognised association with nephrotic syndrome. In the patient described in this scenario, fluid, salt and protein should all be restricted.

Scenario 2

S2.1   A: Unintentional poisoning

The answer here is carbon monoxide poisoning, which is a hard diagnosis to make in clinical practice because of the very vague and non-specific nature of symptoms. Not only can patients present acutely unwell in a coma or with acute mental disturbance, but low-level chronic exposure leads to a clinical picture reminiscent of a viral illness or chronic fatigue, and a careful history is therefore essential.

In this case both the father and his two children are affected, while the mother, who has been away for the last week, has improved away from home, where the source of carbon monoxide is likely to be.

S2.2   E: Commence oxygen therapy

In this family an arterial blood gas, which measures the level of carboxyhaemoglobin, is essential to assess the degree of poisoning. This has to be taken as soon as possible after exposure as carbon monoxide has a half-life of only a few hours and a delayed blood gas will underestimate the extent of poisoning. Most patients can be treated in their local hospital with high-flow oxygen, which shortens the half-life, while those with severe poisoning and in extremis will have to be transferred to the local hyperbaric chamber for treatment.

QUESTIONS ON PAGE 5

Scenario 3

S3.1   E: Intravenous fluids

S3.2   C: Drug interaction

The underlying diagnosis in this patient is rhabdomyolysis leading to acute renal failure, which has been precipitated by the interaction between amiodarone and simvastatin. Amiodarone inhibits cytochrome P450 enzymes and so increases the risk of statin-induced rhabdomyolysis. The urine result hints at this diagnosis by revealing blood + + +, which is due to interference from myoglobin. Patients who are started on amiodarone should be appropriately counselled and care should be taken if they are also on warfarin, theophylline and simvastatin because of the range of interactions.

Scenario 4

S4.1   B: Paget's disease

The description of bone pain and bowing of an extremity are highly suggestive of Paget's disease of the bone and the increased heat is secondary to a high vascular supply to the affected region. In addition to these symptoms, Paget's can also affect the skull, leading to frontal bossing, headaches, hearing loss and trapped nerves.

Paget's disease is a consequence of excessive osteoclastic bone resorption followed by disorganised and uncoordinated osteoblastic bone formation, which leads to weakened and deformed bones. Patients with Paget's disease have a 1% chance of going on to develop sarcoma.

S4.2   E: Osteoclast inhibition

The treatment of choice in Paget's disease is bisphosphonate agents, which inhibit osteoclastic activity and prevent further bone resorption.

QUESTIONS ON PAGE 7

Scenario 5

S5.1 C: Digoxin

This patient has acute on chronic renal failure, as evidenced by the deteriorated creatinine level, which has led to the accumulation of renally excreted drugs such as digoxin and resulted in digoxin toxicity. This is manifested by nausea and vomiting, which might underlie her renal deterioration but which are also non-specific symptoms of digoxin toxicity. More characteristically, she describes xanthopsia, or a yellow tinge to lights and objects. Cardiac manifestations of excess digoxin are bradyarrhythmias, ventricular ectopics, variable degrees of heart block and, rarely, ventricular tachycardia or fibrillation.

S5.2 C: Potassium levels

In patients with digoxin toxicity it is vital to measure potassium levels as hypokalaemia potentiates the cardiac effects of digoxin and even patients with therapeutic digoxin levels can develop toxicity in the context of hypokalaemia.

answers

Scenario 6

Questions on genetics frequently focus on calculating probabilities of disease. This is not to assess your maths skills, but to ensure that you know the pattern of inheritance and are able to apply this knowledge.

S6.1 C: 50%

In this case one partner has sickle cell disease (HbSS) while the other has sickle cell trait (HbAS) and so 50% of their children will have sickle cell trait while 50% will have sickle cell disease.

S6.2 D: 1/60

On first impressions this question seems difficult and created to mislead, but if you break it down into pieces and draw a family pedigree the answer soon becomes apparent:

Mrs Smith's parents

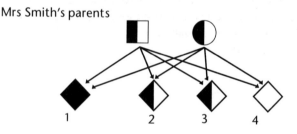

1
2   3
4

Mrs Smith's sibling   Mrs Smith – Carrier or normal?

As Mrs Smith is healthy we know that she is not homozygous for the faulty gene, unlike her brother.

She might be a carrier, for which there are two options: she inherited the faulty gene from her father (2) or she inherited the faulty gene from her mother (3). There is also the possibility that she has a completely normal genotype (4). Her risk for being a carrier is therefore 2/3.

QUESTIONS ON PAGE 9

If we then put all of the facts together:

- The disease is autosomal recessive in its inheritance.
- The risk of Mrs Smith being a carrier is 2/3.
- Mrs Smith's husband carries the population risk of being a carrier, which is 1/10.

The risk of Mrs Smith having an affected child is therefore the risk of Mrs Smith being a carrier × the risk of Mr Smith being a carrier × the risk of having a child with both recessive genes, which we know in autosomal recessive inheritance is 25%, so:

$$2/3 \times 1/10 \times 1/4 = 1/60$$

S6.3 C: Has full penetrance in offspring

Huntingdon's disease is an autosomal dominant triplet repeat disease affecting chromosome 4. The triplet repeat in question is CAG, with the severity of disease dependent on the number of repeats. The disease usually presents in middle-aged patients with movement disorders (chorea) and progresses to seizures, dementia and death. Tetrabenazine can be used to help with movement disturbances but there is currently no treatment that can prevent progression of disease. Encapatone is a COMT inhibitor used in the treatment of Parkinson's disease.

answers

Scenario 7

This patient is presenting with features of hyperosmolar non-ketotic (HONK) coma, (now also known as a hyperosmolar hyperglycaemic state), an emergency occurring in people with type 2 diabetes. It has a high mortality and therefore needs to be taken extremely seriously. For many patients, as in this case, HONK coma can be the first presentation of type 2 diabetes to healthcare services.

S7.1   D: 346

Plasma osmolality = 2 × (sodium + potassium) + urea + glucose

Normal plasma osmolality is between 280 and 310 mosmol/kg.

S7.2   E: Saline fluid administration

High blood glucose levels lead to an osmotic diuresis, accounting for a significant loss of body water. The most important measure is therefore fluid resuscitation using crystalloids such as 0.9% saline or 0.45% saline as opposed to colloids such as Haemaccel or Gelofusine.

After this, a gradual reduction in blood glucose should be achieved using an insulin sliding scale, usually specifically designed for the management of HONK because patients suffering from HONK are usually more sensitive to the effects of insulin compared with patients with diabetic ketoacidosis (DKA).

Intramuscular glucagon is used in patients suffering from hypoglycaemia to raise blood glucose concentrations and is not used in HONK coma.

S7.3   D: In any patient a blood glucose of 7.9 mmol/l 2 hours following an oral glucose tolerance test implies impaired glucose tolerance

If symptomatic (polyuria, polydipsia) then only ONE of the following tests needs to be positive to diagnose type 2 diabetes:

– Random blood glucose > 11.1 mmol/l

OR

– Fasting blood glucose > 7.0 mmol/l

OR

– 2-hour post oral glucose tolerance test blood glucose > 11.1 mmol/l

If the patient is asymptomatic one of the above tests has to be carried out on two separate occasions for a diagnosis to be reached.

A fasting glucose between 6.1 and 7.0 mmol/l implies impaired fasting glycaemia.

A fasting glucose less than 7.0 mmol/l and oral glucose tolerance test between 7.8 and 11.1 mmol/l implies impaired glucose tolerance.

The oral glucose tolerance test is usually reserved for borderline or complex cases.

Although HbA1c is useful for monitoring longer-term blood glucose control, it plays no part in the diagnosis. Good diabetic control aims at keeping HbA1c at less than 7%.

Scenario 8

This patient is suffering from metastatic breast cancer involving the spine and ribs and presents with the common but life-threatening oncological emergency of hypercalcaemia. Within the hospital setting hypercalcaemia is most commonly secondary to malignant disease.

S8.1   D: Bendroflumethiazide

Treatment of hypercalcaemia can include fluid rehydration, loop diuretics, bisphosphonates, steroids, salmon calcitonin and chemotherapy.

In clinical practice intravenous fluids are the first-line agent used to treat hypercalcaemia, both rehydrating the patient and helping to lower the calcium levels. This is combined with the co-administration of bisphosphonates such as pamidronate, which exert their maximal effect 5–7 days after administration.

Thiazide diuretics are avoided because they increase serum calcium levels further.

S8.2   A: Shortened QT interval

Hypercalcaemia causes a shortened QT interval and hypocalcaemia causes a prolonged QT interval. J waves occur in hypothermia and U waves in hypokalaemia.

S8.3   B: Approximately 1500 lives are saved annually by the NHS breast screening programme in the UK

All women registered at general practices between the ages of 50 and 70 are routinely invited for breast cancer screening. Above the age of 70, women are not routinely invited for screening but can attend, free of charge, if they so choose.

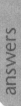

Triple assessment is the method used to assess for breast disease and includes history and examination, imaging and histology/cytology. Younger patients are not suitable for mammography due to increased breast density and therefore ultrasound is the preferred imaging modality in this age group.

HER2 is a proto-oncogene which is targeted by trastuzumab (Herceptin), while tamoxifen is a selective oestrogen antagonist.

Scenario 9

This patient is suffering from bacterial meningitis. Hip flexion in response to passive neck flexion is Brudzinski's sign. Kernig's sign also occurs in meningitis and is elicited by passively flexing the hip with the knee bent – any attempt to straighten the knee causes pain and hamstring spasm.

S9.1   C: Alpha-haemolytic streptococci

The most common organism implicated in meningitis in the elderly is *Streptococcus pneumoniae,* which is an alpha-haemolytic streptococcus.

S9.2   E: Ceftriaxone

A cephalosporin such as ceftriaxone is first-line treatment in patients with streptococcal meningitis. Benzylpenicillin would be more appropriate if *Neisseria meningitidis* was suspected.

S9.3   B: India ink staining of CSF

Cryptococcal meningitis is diagnosed using India ink staining of the CSF, although cryptococcal antigen detection in the CSF can also be used. *Cryptococcus* meningitis is the most common presentation of *Cryptococcus* infection in those who are HIV-positive.

S9.4   B: Renal function tests

Patients with *Cryptococcus* meningitis are usually treated with intravenous amphotericin B, which, although effective, is also nephrotoxic. If renal function is not satisfactory or side-effects of amphotericin B become troublesome, intravenous fluconazole can be used instead.

Scenario 10

This patient appears to have the signs and symptoms of systemic lupus erythematosus (SLE), although the recent introduction of medication strongly supports a diagnosis of drug-induced lupus.

S10.1 A: Isoniazid

Although all of the drugs listed are used in the treatment of *Mycobacterium tuberculosis*, the most likely to cause drug-induced lupus is isoniazid. Isoniazid can also cause a peripheral neuropathy and, although this is rare, patients are started on pyridoxine (vitamin B6) as prophylaxis.

Rifampicin famously alters the colour of body secretions to pink/ orange and in addition it induces liver enzymes, thus reducing the efficacy of other drugs. Female patients on the oral contraceptive pill should be informed of the decreased efficacy and advised to use alternative contraceptive measures.

Pyrazinamide can precipitate hyperuricaemic gout and is also hepatotoxic.

Ethambutol affects vision and all patients started on it should be seen by an ophthalmologist prior to initiation. The earliest indication of visual disturbance is colour blindness for green.

S10.2 E: Anti-histone antibody

In drug-induced SLE anti-histone antibody is present in 90% of patients, although this is not specific for the condition. Anti-nuclear antibody is positive in 50% of patients as opposed to 95% of patients with idiopathic SLE.

S10.3 C: C-reactive protein

In SLE the erythrocyte sedimentation rate is classically raised while C-reactive protein levels can stay normal and therefore CRP is also not as useful as the other investigations to monitor disease activity and progression.

Scenario 11

This patient presents with the triad of weight loss, abdominal pain and diarrhoea, which commonly occurs in Crohn's disease. This is supported by his constitutional symptoms and anal skin tags.

S11.1   D: Azathioprine

Azathioprine takes a number of months to exert its anti-inflammatory effect and therefore has a limited role in the acute management of Crohn's disease, though it can be started at the time of an acute flare of Crohn's.

S11.2   A: Rose-thorn ulceration on sigmoidoscopy

Rose-thorn ulceration is seen on barium studies and not at sigmoidoscopy.

Transmural granulomatous inflammation occurs in Crohn's whereas superficial mucosal ulceration occurs in ulcerative colitis. As inflammation is transmural it allows fistula formation between adjacent anatomical structures such as bowel and skin (enterocutaneous) and bowel and bladder (colovesical).

Both ulcerative colitis and Crohn's disease can be complicated by osteomalacia and by toxic dilatation of the colon, which is a surgical emergency.

S11.3   D: Venous thrombosis

There are numerous extra-gastrointestinal manifestations of inflammatory bowel disease that occur in both ulcerative colitis and Crohn's disease, such as uveitis, conjunctivitis, arthritis, pyoderma gangrenosum and erythema nodosum. Some occur primarily in Crohn's, such as gallstones and renal stones due to the area of bowel affected, while patients with ulcerative colitis are more likely to develop primary sclerosing cholangitis and venous thromboses.

Scenario 12

S12.1   E: Blood pressure of 90/60 mmHg

Hypotension is a feature of life-threatening, not severe asthma.

The parameters for diagnosing a severe asthma attack are:

– Peak expiratory flow rate of between 30% and 50% of expected

– Respiratory rate greater than 25 breaths/minute

– Tachycardia: heart rate > 100 beats per minute

– Inability to complete sentences with one breath

The parameters of life-threatening asthma are:

– Peak expiratory flow rate of < 33% of best or predicted

– Silent chest

– Exhaustion

– Hypotension

– Bradycardia

– Coma

– Rising $PaCO_2$

A useful aid to memory to remember the features of life-threatening asthma is **BREATH**:

Bradycardia

Rising $PaCO_2$

Exhaustion

Absent breath sounds (silent chest)

Third of expected peak flow and GCS of 3 (coma)

Hypotension

Although the student states that he was not able to perform peak flow measurement this is not uncommon during an asthma attack. If his peak flow was < 30% of expected, this would be in keeping with a life-threatening asthma attack.

answers

S12.2 C: Terbutaline 10 mg nebulised

In the management of asthma, patients should be sitting upright in bed and receiving 100% oxygen. Salbutamol is given at a dose of 5 mg nebulised, not 500 micrograms. Ipratropium bromide and steroids should then be considered.

S12.3 A: Asthma affects over 5 million children in the UK

Asthma affects over 5 million individuals in the UK. Approximately 1 million children are affected. All of the other statements are true.

S12.4 B: The medication is known to cause hypokalaemia

The medication is most likely to be a selective ß2-agonist such as salbutamol, which leads to a tremor, palpitations, headaches and hypokalaemia at high doses. Washing the mouth after administration of inhaled steroids is recommended, no matter what dose is given. Atrovent is the trade name for ipratropium bromide, which is more useful in chronic obstructive pulmonary disease than in asthma, although it can be used in an acute asthma attack.

For further information the British Thoracic Society Guidelines are extremely useful and are available online at http://www.brit-thoracic.org.uk/

QUESTIONS ON PAGES 19–20

Scenario 13

An examiner's favourite is the travelling businessman who invariably presents with a sexually transmitted disease (STD).

S13.1   A: *Neisseria gonorrhoeae*

With symptoms of dysuria and profuse discharge the most likely organism is *Neisseria gonorrhoeae*, for which humans are the only host. Despite the above presentation 50% of females and 10% of males are asymptomatic.

S13.2   E: Gram-negative diplococci

N. gonorrhoeae are intracellular Gram-negative diplococci and can be readily seen on microscopy.

S13.3   A: Co-existent infection

It is likely that this patient who has already been treated has an underlying STD in addition to *Neisseria gonorrhoeae*, most likely to be *Chlamydia trachomatis*. It is important when reviewing patients with sexually transmitted diseases to screen for carriage of asymptomatic pathogens and to provide treatment accordingly.

S13.4   D: *Chlamydia trachomatis*

The patient has lymphogranuloma venereum, which is caused by certain strains of *Chlamydia* (L1, L2 and L3).

The primary stage is a painless ulcer occurring on the mucosal membrane of the penetrating site (penis, vagina, rectum). The organism then invades into the lymphatic system and lymph nodes, leading to large and multiple buboes and abscesses in the inguinal lymph nodes which then coalesce and discharge. Rectal lymphogranuloma venereum leads to proctocolitis as in this patient and pharyngeal disease can also occur affecting the cervical lymph node chain.

Scenario 14

This patient presents with a compression fracture of her thoracic vertebrae secondary to osteoporosis.

S14.1   B: Myxoedema

The list of causes and precipitating factors for osteoporosis is long but hyperthyroidism, not hypothyroidism, is associated with osteoporosis.

A range of medications can lead to osteoporosis, including steroids, ciclosporin and long-term administration of unfractionated heparin.

S14.2   B: Peak bone mass is attained between the second and third decades of life

Around 95% of peak bone mass is accrued by the age of 18–20 years and rises slightly in the following decade before starting to fall.

Routine blood tests in osteoporosis are usually returned as normal unless there has been a recent fracture. A T-score between −1 and −2.5 represents osteopenia, while a score less than −2.5 represents osteoporosis.

The exaggerated kyphosis limits chest wall movement, leading to a restrictive defect on spirometry and severe kyphosis can lead to type 2 respiratory failure.

The gold-standard investigation for diagnosing osteoporosis is a DEXA scan (dual-energy X-ray absorption scan).

S14.3 D: Osteoporosis is implicated in over 150 000 fractures annually in the UK

Parathyroid hormone increases the level of circulating calcium but decreases the level of phosphate compared with vitamin D, which increases the levels of both calcium and phosphate.

Vitamin D undergoes hydroxylation twice: the first step is carried out by the liver, while the second hydroxylation step (1α-hydroxylation), to form the most active form, is carried out by the kidneys. Patients with chronic kidney disease in whom this function is diminished are therefore prescribed the active form of vitamin D to preserve their bone health.

The dietary recommended values for prevention of osteoporosis include 800–1200 mg of calcium daily and 400–600 IU of vitamin D.

Scenario 15

S15.1   D: Erythema multiforme

This is the characteristic description of erythema multiforme, which in its most severe form can result in widespread blisters on the mucous membranes of the mouth and genitalia – Stevens–Johnson syndrome.

Pyoderma gangrenosum comprises erythematous nodules which ulcerate and spread rapidly with a necrotic-looking leading edge. They are classically associated with inflammatory bowel disease but also occur in haematological malignancies and in other autoimmune disorders.

Erythema nodosum comprises tender, shiny erythematous lesions which classically affect the shins bilaterally and which are caused by inflammation of the subcutaneous fat layer. The most common cause of erythema nodosum is streptococcal infection but it can also occur in tuberculosis and in *Chlamydia* infections. Other key associated diseases are inflammatory bowel disease and sarcoidosis.

Erythema marginatum is a rash associated with rheumatic fever and is the presence of a spreading erythematous maculopapular lesion with central clearing.

Erythema chronicum migrans is the rash typically associated with Lyme disease and is described as a 'bullseye' lesion, with central erythema surrounded by a halo of pale skin, which itself is surrounded by erythema.

S15.2   C: Herpes simplex

The most common identified cause of erythema multiforme is herpes simplex, although in 50% of cases the cause is unknown.

QUESTIONS ON PAGE 26

Scenario 16

The management of hypertension is a very important topic that all students should be familiar with, including which drugs are indicated for which patients for primary treatment and their subsequent side-effects.

S16.1 E: Nifedipine

Nifedipine is a calcium-channel blocker which can cause gum hypertrophy; other side-effects include headaches, flushing and ankle oedema.

S16.2 B: Non-concordance

The patient's blood pressure is not under control because he has not been taking his medication, which in this case is likely to be a beta-blocker, in keeping with the side-effects mentioned.

'Non-concordance' is the best phrase to use as it implies an imbalance between the ideas, concerns and expectations of the doctor and the patient rather than the patient just not following their doctor's advice.

Mullen PD, Compliance becomes concordance: editorial. *BMJ* 1997; 314: 691.

answers

S16.3 D: Ultrasound

This patient with resistant hypertension was most likely started on an ACE inhibitor, which caused a decrease in GFR and renal function, as measured by the Cockcroft–Gault formula. The underlying pathology is therefore most likely to be renal artery stenosis (RAS) and the initial investigation of choice would be an ultrasound to look for a difference in size between the right and left kidney, with a size difference of 2 cm between left and right suggesting RAS. Doppler studies can also be used concurrently to look for evidence of post-stenosis turbulence, raised peak systolic velocities or a raised velocity in the renal artery 3.5 times higher than the abdominal aorta. Any suggestion of RAS can then be followed by magnetic resonance imaging for further detailed information.

S16.4 E: Angiography

The gold-standard imaging technique to diagnose RAS is formal angiography, although, due to the invasive nature of the procedure and the risks of contrast nephropathy, it is not commonly undertaken as a diagnostic tool but more as an interventional tool to correct underlying RAS.

S16.5 A: Losartan

In this patient, the first thing to do is to ensure that the worsening smoker's cough is not a sign of new underling pathology such as cancer and is attributable to the new medication that was started. This patient was started on an ACE inhibitor, which also increase the levels of bradykinin, accounting for the cough. In such cases ACE inhibitors can be substituted with angiotensin II receptor antagonists such as losartan.

Scenario 17

The history of tiredness, slim build, diarrhoea and rash is consistent with coeliac disease or gluten enteropathy.

S17.1   E: Dermatitis herpetiformis

The fax report is consistent with the above diagnosis.

S17.2   A: Non-drug treatment

The first-line treatment of dermatitis herpetiformis and coeliac disease is the exclusion of gluten-containing substances from the diet.

S17.3   D: Glucose-6-phosphate dehydrogenase deficiency

The history is consistent with haemolytic anaemia and suggests the patient has an underlying tendency to develop haemolytic crises. The most commonly inherited enzyme defect is G6PD deficiency, a sex-linked disease in which the sufferers are susceptible to haemolytic anaemia in response to certain drugs and, famously, fava beans.

The patient is likely to have been started on dapsone, which is used both in the treatment of Hansen's disease (leprosy) and dermatitis herpetiformis, and is a known trigger in patients suffering from G6PD deficiency.

answers

Scenario 18

This patient has developed the complication of pseudomembranous colitis due to *Clostridium difficile*, a common occurrence in hospitals that leads to significant distress, delay in discharge, morbidity and mortality.

S18.1   B: Stool toxin analysis

Although *C. difficile* can be cultured, not all strains produce the toxin that causes diarrhoea and therefore it is best to test for the presence of the toxin, which is why the test is also known as CDT (**C**lostridium **d**ifficile **T**oxin).

S18.2   A: Gram-positive rod

S18.3   D: Metronidazole

The treatment of *C. difficile* usually involves oral metronidazole or oral vancomycin. Metronidazole is the preferred first-line agent, followed by vancomycin if not successful.

A key to prevent the spread of *Clostridium difficile* is thorough and careful hand-washing with soap and water before and after seeing patients, as alcohol gel alone does not remove the spores. Additional measures include removing wristwatches and rolling up sleeves.

QUESTIONS ON PAGE 32

Scenario 19

The features are consistent with a diagnosis of cystic fibrosis, a common autosomal recessive genetic disorder. The gene affected is for the cystic fibrosis transmembrane regulator (CFTR), which is a protein that functions as a chloride channel. Abnormalities in chloride secretion lead to viscous fluids and result in excess inflammation and infections due to the impaired clearance of secretions.

S19.1 B: 1/25

The carrier frequency in the white population is approximately 1/20 to 1/25. The actual incidence of the disease is 1/2500 live births.

S19.2 C: *Pseudomonas aeruginosa*

Pseudomonas aeruginosa is a common pathogen found in patients with cystic fibrosis. It is an opportunistic organism, infection usually occurring in immunocompromised and severely ill patients. The green sputum is highly characteristic and occurs due to a blue-green pigment produced by the bacteria.

S19.3 A: Ciprofloxacin

Of the antibiotics listed, ciprofloxacin is the most commonly used oral agent to treat *Pseudomonas aeruginosa*.

Scenario 20

Understanding medical statistics is essential in order to be fully informed about scientific studies, research and novel treatments, and also to enable critical appraisal of product literature and pharmaceutical promotions.

S20.1 A: Case-controlled study

In a case–controlled study subjects who already have the disease (in this case, breast cancer) are compared with controls who do not. Once the cases and controls have been identified, the past exposure to the aetiological agent is analysed (in this case substance X).

A randomised controlled trial is when subjects are randomly allocated to receive treatment A or B (substance X or placebo) and fixed outcomes are measured within a given time-frame. Single-blinded trials are those in which the patients do not know which treatment group they are in but researchers do. In double-blinded studies both the researchers and patients are unaware of which treatment is being given. Under certain circumstances it is impossible to blind trials.

A cohort study is an example of a longitudinal analysis. An example of a cohort study is as follows: 50 patients who are exposed to substance X (for example) would be studied alongside 50 patients who were not, to look for complications and the occurrence of breast cancer. In real life, longitudinal studies involve many hundreds or thousands of patients followed up over many years or decades.

S20.2 E: 2 standard deviations

If data are normally distributed, then 2 standard deviations from the mean includes 95% of the population. The remaining 5% are a split of the upper 2.5% and lower 2.5%.

S20.3 C: Echocardiography

The gold-standard investigation to assess heart failure and ventricular function is echocardiography.

S20.4 A: 83%

Sensitivity can be defined as the percentage of people testing positive for the disease out of all of those who actually have the disease.

Specificity can be defined as the percentage of people who tested negative for the disease out of all of those without the disease.

It is always useful to tabulate the information as below:

		Heart Failure	
		Present	Absent
Blood Test	Positive	250	50
	Negative	50	150

In the above example 250 people tested positive on the blood test who actually had the disease out of a total of 300 (250 + 50).

Therefore the sensitivity is 250/300 × 100 = 83%

Scenario 21

S21.1 B: Ultrasound

In a patient with acute renal failure it is vital to conduct an appropriate history and examination and from the list given the ultrasound scan is least useful in the initial assessment and treatment, although it is vital in the subsequent investigations to exclude an obstructive nephropathy.

S21.2 D: 50% dextrose with 10 units Actrapid insulin

This patient has hyperkalaemia, evident from the ECG changes described. Urgent IV access should be established, with blood taken for biochemistry to measure how high the potassium is. The patient should be given calcium gluconate or calcium chloride which act to stabilise heart muscle from arrhythmias.

However, to correct the underlying abnormality, dextrose and insulin, salbutamol and, in extremely severe cases dialysis are needed to reduce serum potassium concentrations.

QUESTIONS ON PAGE 37

Scenario 22

The management of patients suffering cardiac or respiratory arrest should be memorised using the new guidelines for basic and advanced life support.

S22.1 D: 30 compressions to 2 breaths

Recommendations suggest 30 compressions to 2 breaths.

S22.2 D: Defibrillate at 360 J

Recommendations suggest one shock at 360 joules.

S22.3 D: Resume CPR for 2 minutes

Recommendations suggest that after one shock CPR should be re-started for a further 2 minutes and medication given.

S22.4 B: Atropine

In this case the bradycardia guidelines should be put into place, which suggest atropine as a first-line agent.

S22.5 B: Transcutaneous pacing

Failure to respond to atropine and a deteriorating patient requires urgent transcutaneous pacing until transvenous pacing can be established.

All of the above guidelines and other useful information and resources can be accessed from the Resuscitation Council (UK) website: www.resus.org.uk

Scenario 23

Paracetamol (acetaminophen) is the most common drug overdose in the UK and is potentially life-threatening. Accurate knowledge about its management is therefore essential.

S23.1 D: Activated charcoal is better than gastric lavage in this situation

The hepatotoxic dose of paracetamol for most patients is 150 mg/kg but those who are at high risk secondary to reduced glutathione reserves can develop severe hepatic failure with much lower blood paracetamol levels. Paracetamol overdose leads to approximately 200 deaths per year and N-acetylcysteine is almost 100% successful in preventing significant hepatic impairment if used within 8 hours.

S23.2 D: Methionine is an alternative to N-acetylcysteine

High-risk patients are those in whom glutathione reserves are diminished and include patients with anorexia nervosa. Approximately 10% of patients report an allergic reaction to N-acetylcysteine, occasionally leading to anaphylaxis, and methionine is a useful secondary agent. The prothrombin time is the best indicator for severity of liver disease in paracetamol overdoses.

S23.3 D: Cimetidine

When deciding who to treat with N-acetylcysteine you first need to risk-stratify patients into high or low risk. Those who are high-risk need treatment if their paracetamol levels are above the lower treatment line on the charts. Those found not to be at high risk require treatment if paracetamol levels are above the higher treatment line. Patients at high risk include those with HIV (irrespective of whether they are on HAART), people with anorexia nervosa and people on enzyme-inducing drugs such as phenytoin and carbamazepine. Cimetidine does not deplete glutathione so users who take a paracetamol overdose are not counted as high-risk.

S23.4 B: Prothrombin time the same as the control

The prothrombin time is used to calculate the international normalised ratio (INR). The INR is a good marker for hepatic dysfunction due to paracetamol toxicity and is therefore useful in assessing the severity. In serious paracetamol overdoses the INR can rise to above 5 and therefore an INR of 1, which is what this statement implies, is reassuring.

Scenario 24

This lady presents with a significant smoking history, weight loss and haemoptysis, so a neoplasm should be the main differential.

S24.1 C: Chest X-ray

A PA chest X-ray is the most important initial investigation and would detect suspicious soft-tissue densities. This is especially useful given the long smoking history and sinister features mentioned in the scenario.

S24.2 A: 0.9% saline for 12 hours prior to the procedure

This lady has pre-existing renal impairment as shown by the raised urea and creatinine and is also on metformin for her diabetes. She is therefore at great risk of developing contrast-induced nephropathy. This is often not taken into consideration when people have CT scans with contrast. It presents as acute deterioration in renal function secondary to the contrast medium used and can lead to significant morbidity and mortality.

Good hydration prior to and following the procedure helps minimise the risk, as does stopping metformin 48 hours before the scan. A number of agents are used in an attempt to prevent contrast-induced nephropathy, including N-acetylcysteine, aminophylline and statins.

Contrast-induced nephropathy is also of concern in people undergoing interventional radiological procedures and coronary angiography. Renal function should be monitored in these people following the investigation.

QUESTIONS ON PAGES 42–43

Scenario 25

This patient presents with acute pancreatitis secondary to alcohol. Pancreatitis is a surgical emergency that often arises in exams.

S25.1 D: Measles

Mumps but not measles is a risk factor for developing pancreatitis.

S25.2 A: Amylase

Although amylase is useful in the diagnosis of pancreatitis, it is not useful for the assessment of severity. A useful mnemonic to aid in memorising the severity of pancreatitis is **PANCREAS**:

PaO_2 < 8 kPa

Age > 55

Neutrophils > 15 × 10^9/l

Corrected calcium < 2 mmol/l

Raised urea > 15 mmol/l

Elevated LDH > 600 IU

Albumin < 30 g/l

Sugar (BM) < 10 mmol

If three or more of the above criteria are satisfied, an attack of pancreatitis is labelled as severe. The above features make up the Glasgow Criteria, which are only valid after 24–48 hours after onset of pancreatitis. Alternative severity scores such as APACHE II can be used prior to 24 hours.

S25.3 C: Enteral nutrition is of benefit in patients with this condition

Patients with pancreatitis are usually very ill and will require nutritional support to aid their recovery. This is most needed in those with severe disease, with the enteral route being preferred due to lower costs and side-effects.

If pancreatitis is thought to be secondary to gallstones, then urgent ERCP should be performed, ideally less than 72 hours after presentation.

UK Guidelines for the management of acute pancreatitis: *Gut* 2005; 54: 1–9.

QUESTION ON PAGES 44–45

Scenario 26

A common problem in all hospitals is the treatment of alcohol withdrawal and its complications.

S26.1 D: Chlordiazepoxide

Chlordiazepoxide is the benzodiazepine of choice in the management of alcohol withdrawal as it has a longer period of action and a less marked withdrawal response. In patients with significant liver disease lorazepam is preferred.

S26.2 A: Insulin

Fluid rehydration, intravenous thiamine and B vitamins and benzodiazepines form the cornerstone of treatment. Patients are at risk of developing hypoglycaemia and so insulin is not routinely indicated in these patients. Hypophosphataemia is another complication which may require supplementation.

S26.3 C: Wernicke syndrome is the triad of ophthalmoplegia, nystagmus and amnesia

Wernicke syndrome is the triad of ophthalmoplegia and nystagmus, ataxia and encephalopathy (acute mental confusion).

Amnesia would be more in keeping with Korsakoff syndrome – a progression of Wernicke's encephalopathy.

answers

Scenario 27

Patients in nursing homes who are immobile for long periods of time are susceptible to developing sigmoid volvulus, as in this case, in which a loop of bowel twists round itself, leading to absolute obstruction and constipation, abdominal distension and pain. It is more common in those who are constipated.

S27.1 A: Abdominal X-ray

An abdominal X-ray would show the characteristic coffee-bean sign of large-bowel obstruction of the sigmoid colon. The large bowel can become very distended due to a closed loop system and there is a significant risk of perforation.

S27.2 D: Sigmoid volvulus

See above.

S27.3 D: Flatus tube insertion

Conservative management of flatus tube insertion or flexible sigmoidoscopy can be all that is required to relieve the obstruction and untwist the bowel. Occasionally, more aggressive surgical treatment is required.

QUESTIONS ON PAGE 48

Scenario 28

The extremely high white cell count, hepatomegaly and splenomegaly point towards a diagnosis of leukaemia. The t(9:22) translocation, known as the Philadelphia chromosome, is a common genetic abnormality seen in chronic myeloid leukaemia. The t(9:22) translocation leads to the creation of the *BCR-ABL* gene, an oncogene with tyrosine kinase activity.

S28.1 C: Philadelphia chromosome

See above.

S28.2 A: Chronic myeloid leukaemia

See above.

S28.3 A: Imatinib mesylate

Imatinib mesylate, also known as Gleevec, is a tyrosine kinase inhibitor and blocks the action of the *BCR-ABL* gene. It is also useful in the treatment of certain stromal tumours.

answers

Scenario 29

This patient is likely to have bleeding oesophageal varices, a medical emergency because of the large volume of blood that can be lost.

S29.1 E: Terlipressin

Terlipressin has been shown to decrease mortality by causing splanchnic vasoconstriction and is preferred over vasopressin.

S29.2 C: Propranolol

Beta-blockers such as propranolol are useful for decreasing the risk of re-bleeding and all patients with established varices or developing hypertensive changes should be considered for propranolol.

QUESTIONS ON PAGE 50

SECTION 2: KNOWLEDGE-BASED ANSWERS

K1   C: Diabetic ketoacidosis typically has an onset of less than 24 hours

Diabetic ketoacidosis (DKA) and hyperosmolar hyperglycaemic states (the new name for hyperosmolar non-ketotic coma) are two of the main diabetic emergencies, and arise as a result of the metabolic complications of sustained hyperglycaemia.

Diabetic ketoacidosis can occur in patients with either type 1 or type 2 diabetes mellitus but is relatively more common in type 1 diabetes and therefore affects younger individuals. The most common precipitating factor is an infection, usually urinary tract in origin. However, note that a raised white cell count can be a finding in patients with DKA without any underlying infection. DKA tends to evolve within 1 day while hyperosmolar states develop over a few days. The mortality rate of DKA is nearly 5%, whereas for hyperosmolar hyperglycaemic states the mortality lies between 15% and 25%.

K2   C: ECG

The patient has a diagnosis of a pulmonary embolism, given the sudden onset of shortness of breath, haemoptysis and hypoxia, caused by a recent hip operation and prolonged immobility. Given the high pre-test probability of a pulmonary embolism, a D-dimer test should not be performed because, regardless of the result, you will investigate with a CT pulmonary angiogram or a ventilation-perfusion scan to confirm your clinical suspicion. The place of D-dimer testing is in those patients with a low pre-test probability of a pulmonary embolism and to help in its exclusion. D-Dimers should not be used for diagnostic reasons because although the sensitivity of the test is high, the specificity is low.

A bronchoscopy is not useful as the haemoptysis does not reflect an underlying suspicion of malignancy or infection. A low-grade pyrexia is a common finding in patients with a pulmonary embolism and blood cultures are therefore not the most appropriate investigation. In the acute setting, a PA or an AP chest X-ray is vital in the acute assessment of a patient with shortness of breath, but a lateral X-ray would not be required.

The most appropriate investigation is therefore an ECG.

200

QUESTION ON PAGE 52

K3 **D: Aldosterone is secreted from the zona glomerulosa of the adrenal cortex and affects sodium and potassium homeostasis, particularly in the distal tubule of the kidney**

Prolactin is under negative feedback from dopamine released by the anterior pituitary and therefore prolactin levels are raised in patients on dopamine agonists. Dopamine agonists include bromocriptine, cabergoline and pramipexole.

Cortisol secretion is indeed diurnal, but with highest levels occurring between 8 and 9am and lowest levels occurring at midnight. This is why cortisol samples are usually taken in the morning and labelled '9am cortisol levels'.

In response to renal hypoperfusion the kidneys secrete renin, which cleaves angiotensinogen to angiotensin I. This is then cleaved by angiotensin-converting enzyme found within the lung to the highly active form of angiotensin II.

LH stimulates the production of testosterone from Leydig cells while FSH stimulates the production of mature sperm by acting on the Sertoli cells.

K4 C: Confusion is a risk factor in the development of pressure sores

Pressure sores are a very common and serious problem in nursing home residents as well as in hospital inpatients. Not only do they cause significant morbidity but they also represent a huge burden on the NHS and as with nearly everything in medicine, prevention is better than cure.

Screening should be undertaken on admission to identify not only those with active pressure sores but those who are at high risk for developing them. Based on this, appropriate interventions can be undertaken such as regular turning, use of a pressure-relieving mattress, surgical involvement and so on. Early tissue viability nurse assessment is vital for improving patient care and moist occlusive dressings are useful in the treatment of pressure sores.

The European Pressure Ulcer Advisory Panel classification system of pressure ulcer grades:

– Grade 1: non-blanching erythema of intact skin. In individuals with darker skins, discoloration of the skin, warmth, oedema, induration or hardness can also be used as indicators.

– Grade 2: partial-thickness skin loss involving epidermis or dermis, or both. The ulcer is superficial and presents clinically as an abrasion or blister.

– Grade 3: full-thickness skin loss involving damage to or necrosis of subcutaneous tissue that can extend down to, but not through, underlying fascia.

– Grade 4: extensive destruction, tissue necrosis, or damage to muscle, bone or supporting structures with or without full-thickness skin loss.

Further information: NICE guidelines on the management of pressure ulcers, available from http://www.nice.org.uk/guidance/CG29

QUESTION ON PAGE 53

K5   B: Aplastic anaemia

The patient presents with severe anaemia, leukopenia and thrombocytopenia, with a hypoplastic marrow, and the most likely diagnosis is aplastic anaemia. Myelodysplastic syndrome is a disease of the elderly, with decreasing production and quality of blood components. Evans syndrome is the presence of autoimmune haemolysis and autoimmune thrombocytopenia together in the same patient.

K6   E: βhCG estimation

Although the history for this patient is suggestive of polycystic ovary disease, it is extremely important to exclude pregnancy in any patient presenting with amenorrhoea before considering alternative diagnoses.

K7   D: Red blood cells sensitised in vivo to autoantibodies can be detected using the direct Coombs' reaction

Haemolytic disease of the newborn usually occurs in the context of rhesus disease, in which a rhesus-negative mother is sensitised to her rhesus-positive baby in the first pregnancy. In subsequent pregnancies the IgG antibodies made by the mother can cross the placenta, leading to haemolysis.

Goodpasture's disease is an example of type II hypersensitivity, where antibodies cause damage by binding to their antigen in tissues. Type III hypersensitivity is caused by immune complex deposition. Anaphylactic reactions are triggered by IgE antibodies, not IgA. HIV uses CXCR4 and CCR5 as co-receptors for entry into CD4+ T cells.

K8   D: Aspiration of synovial fluid

In a patient with a temperature and joint pain the most important disease process to rule out is septic arthritis. The most appropriate investigation is therefore aspiration of synovial fluid for culture, sensitivity and microscopy, although a full septic screen should always be undertaken. The patient should be started on appropriate antibiotics as soon as possible to avoid long-term damage to the joint.

K9   B: Hepatitis B virus

All of the others are examples of RNA viruses.

K10   A: ST depression and tall R waves in leads V1 and V2 is consistent with a posterior myocardial infarction

The corrected QT interval = QT interval / square root of the RR interval.

Low-voltage QRS complexes are caused by things such as hypothyroidism, COPD and increased haemocrit, but not obesity.

This question is about choosing the answer that is *most right* as although S1Q3T3 can occur with pulmonary emboli, it is not a common finding.

A finding of 2-mm ST elevation in leads II, III, aVF, V4 and V5 suggests an inferior-lateral infarction as opposed to just an inferior myocardial infarction.

K11 E: The Trendelenburg test is useful for assessing the competence of the sapheno-femoral junction

As the long saphenous is a vein its course is from distal to proximal, therefore statement A is false. The sapheno-femoral junction is 4 cm inferior and lateral to the pubic tubercle. The profunda femoris is an artery within the thigh that is a branch of the femoral artery. It is therefore not used in coronary artery bypass grafting, as opposed to the long saphenous vein. A saphena varix classically transmits a cough impulse and disappears when the patient is asked to lie down.

K12 D: Small-bowel ischaemia

The triad of severe acute abdominal pain, severe shock and a lack of significant abdominal findings points to a diagnosis of small-bowel ischaemia. We know that the patient is an arteriopath with a previous myocardial infarction and the 'heartburn' after eating is probably mesenteric ischaemia of the gut due to atherosclerosis. The patient has developed a thrombus within the mesenteric circulation, leading to small-bowel ischaemia and the presentation described.

K13 D: Work with colleagues in a way which best serves the health service

The statement should read: 'Work with colleagues in a way which best serves patients.'

Further information from the General Medical Council website: http://www.gmc-uk.org/

K14   C: The combined oral contraceptive pill can be used to treat acne vulgaris

In female patients who have failed treatment with oral antibiotics and require a form of contraception, the combined oral contraceptive pill is a useful agent provided there are no contraindications such as breast cancer, an age of greater than 35 while smoking more than 15 cigarettes a day, migraines with aura, or previous deep vein thrombosis.

Condoms have a success approaching 98%–99% when used correctly, while the rates of failure of female tubal ligation are considerably worse than the failure rate of vasectomy in men.

K15   C: Pernicious anaemia

The patient has a megaloblastic anaemia due to vitamin B12 deficiency and subsequent neuropathy. These features combined with the sore mouth and looser stool is suggestive of pernicious anaemia.

QUESTIONS ON PAGE 59

K16 A: Nodular melanoma is a highly aggressive form of the disease

Melanoma is a malignancy of melanocytes, with a major causative factor being exposure to ultraviolet radiation during childhood and adolescence. Nodular melanoma is the most aggressive form of the disease and invades vertically early and grows rapidly. Superficial spreading melanoma, as its name suggests, usually exhibits lateral spread followed by vertical spread. Breslow thickness is the depth of tumour invasion and is measured from the surface to the area of deepest penetration of the skin and is a more reliable prognostic marker than Clark's level, which describes which layer the melanoma cells have infiltrated to. Patients with metastatic disease have an extremely poor prognosis of between 5%–15% at 5 years and this is the reason why education, prevention and early detection and treatment are vital.

The **ABCDE criteria** for worrying signs in a mole:

Asymmetry of the mole

Border irregularity

Colour variegation

Diameter greater than 6 mm

Elevation or enlarging mole

answers

K17 E: *Streptococcus pneumoniae*

The patient has presented with a simple community-acquired pneumonia and the bronchial breathing and the rust-coloured sputum point towards a diagnosis of *Streptococcus pneumoniae*. The recent trip to Spain with his friends might raise the suspicion of *Legionella* but the question does not give enough information to confirm this diagnosis (typical features are fevers with dry cough, myalgia, liver dysfunction and hyponatraemia).

The other red herring is that the patient is an abattoir worker and could be at risk of Q fever due to *Coxiella burnetii* but again there is not enough information to support this diagnosis in the form of a severe flu-like illness with myalgia, severe headache and excessive perspiration.

K18 C: Post-exposure prophylaxis is indicated in high-risk cases only

The seroconversion rate from needlestick injuries in which the patient is known to have HIV is 0.4% while the risk of developing hepatitis B or C from a similar needlestick injury is much higher (30%–60%). Exposure through mucous membranes carries a lower risk than through penetrating injuries with needles.

The doctor should safely stop what he is doing and wash and bleed his thumb under running water. After this he should present himself to the Occupational Health Department which will offer HIV counselling and negotiate taking blood and testing the patient in question. If Occupational Health is closed the doctor should present himself to the Emergency Department, where the on-call virologist can make the decision on whether to start post-exposure prophylaxis.

Patients who are at low risk, either due to the nature of the incident or the patient (HIV-negative and/or no risk factors) do not need post-exposure prophylaxis (PEP).

QUESTIONS ON PAGES 60–61

K19 B: Amenorrhoea often precedes weight loss

The patient is suffering from anorexia nervosa, which is an eating disorder more common than was initially thought and extremely difficult to treat. Although more common in females, one out of ten sufferers will be male and, unlike most medical conditions, those in higher socioeconomic groups are more affected. A BMI of less than 17.5 kg/m^2 or a weight less than 85% of that predicted is classically used to define anorexia.

K20   D: Only people with parental responsibility are allowed to give consent on behalf of children

For consent to be valid, three main principles have to be met. Firstly the patient must have been appropriately informed about the procedure, the benefits and disadvantages of undertaking the proposed treatment, and the various other treatment options available, including the consequences of having no treatment. Secondly, the consent has to be freely given, without coercion from doctors, relatives or friends. (Although the medical team can advise patients and guide them in their choice, they should not abuse their position.) Finally, the patient must be competent to make that decision, which does not require them to be able to read and write.

Consent for procedures can only be undertaken by the consultant undertaking the procedure or by a different consultant, registrar or doctor who has sufficient experience with the same procedure. In some cases, appropriately trained healthcare personnel can also be trained to take consent, such as nurse specialists in endoscopy.

Patients should be told about commonly occurring risks, especially those with a frequency of greater than 1%, but also should be told about rarer complications which might have a profound effect on that patient. For example, even if the risk of blindness of an operation was 1 in 20 000, given the severity of the complication a patient would be within their rights to know about that risk when weighing up their final decision. There have been many cases of patients who develop a rare complication after treatment who have successfully sued the consultant on the basis of not being appropriately informed and consented.

In the case of children, only those adults with parental responsibility can give valid consent on behalf of the child and this includes the mother, the father if he was married to the mother at the time of conception or if the biological father marries the mother at a later date, and adults who have legally adopted a child or who have got a court order issuing them with parental responsibility.

Further information on consent and capacity is available from the General Medical Council, the Medical Defence Union or the Medical Protection Society.

QUESTION ON PAGE 63

K21 E: Immobility is a contraindication to treatment with the disease-modifying beta-interferon medications

Multiple sclerosis usually presents as a relapsing-remitting disease in 85% of cases as opposed to primary progressive multiple sclerosis. Half of those with relapsing-remitting disease will go on to develop secondary progressive disease.

The risk of multiple sclerosis increases the further from the equator you grow up, and those people who emigrate after adolescence carry the risk of their original country. A sibling's risk of developing multiple sclerosis is between 2% and 5%, which is much higher than in the general population.

Optic neuritis is a common presentation of multiple sclerosis but normal optic discs are usually seen in retrobulbar neuritis prior to the occurrence of optic atrophy, which develops over days to weeks.

Oligoclonal bands in the CSF which are *not* matched in the serum are highly suggestive of multiple sclerosis but are not pathognomonic of multiple sclerosis.

Indications for treatment with newer disease-modifying drugs in multiple sclerosis include:

- Relapsing-remitting multiple sclerosis

- Ability to walk independently with or without assistance

- Age > 17 years

- Two clinically significant attacks within 2 years

- No major contraindications (see *BNF*)

answers

QUESTION ON PAGE 63

K22   D: The features are consistent with sodium valproate treatment

The side-effects of sodium valproate can be remembered using the mnemonic **WHAAT**:

Weight gain

Hyperammonaemia (including nausea, vomiting and malaise)

Ankle swelling

Ataxia and tremor

Thinning hair

K23   E: Weight loss

Irritable bowel syndrome is a complex disease that has a range of symptoms, all of which are listed in the question, apart from weight loss, which is most suggestive of an underlying organic cause.

K24   E: Randomised controlled trial

When assessing the relationship between two variables the best method to use is a double-blinded randomised controlled trial.

K25   A: Tropicamide

Tropicamide and cyclopentolate are both mydriatics, the former being short-acting, the latter long-acting. Pilocarpine is a miotic agent and tetracaine is a local anaesthetic agent.

QUESTIONS ON PAGES 64-65

K26   A: Sjögren syndrome

The presence of rheumatoid factor, an IgM (rarely IgG) antibody whose Fab portion binds the Fc portion of immunoglobulins occurs in a range of autoimmune diseases. The incidence in rheumatoid arthritis increases with increasing disease duration, being present in approximately 70%–80% of individuals.

The presence of rheumatoid factor is much higher in Felty syndrome and in Sjögren syndrome.

K27   C: Chondrosarcoma

Cotton-wool calcification is seen typically with chondrosarcoma, while sunray spiculation and Codman's triangle occur in osteosarcoma.

K28   B: Delusional perceptions

Schneiderian first-rank symptoms include:

1. Auditory hallucinations:

    a.   Voices speaking the patient's thoughts aloud

    b.   Voices describing the patient's activity

    c.   Voices arguing amongst themselves about the patient

2. Delusional perception: patients take a normal perception (such as seeing a bird on a tree) but interpret it abnormally (such as believing it to be a sign that the aliens are coming)

3. Somatic hallucinations

4. Thought insertion/withdrawal/broadcast

5. Control of affect by outside forces

6. Control of action by outside forces

Although Schneiderian first-rank symptoms are not pathognomonic of schizophrenia they are useful to remember for exams and when reviewing patients.

answers

K29 C: Left homonymous scotoma – right occipital cortex

Bitemporal hemianopia occurs with a lesion of the optic chiasm. Superior quadrantanopia occurs with temporal lesions, inferior quadrantanopia with parietal lesions. Monocular anopia occurs with damage to the optic nerve.

If the occipital lobe is affected at the tip it is possible for only the central vision to be affected, producing a scotoma, while the peripheral vision will be relatively unaffected. However, if the entire occipital lobe is affected, then a homonymous hemianopia would occur.

K30 D: Pterygium

A degenerative yellow nodule on the conjunctiva either side of the cornea is known as a 'pinguecula'. These can sometimes encroach onto the cornea, when they become known as 'pterygium', typically occurring in dusty and wind-blown areas.

Hordeolum is the fancy name for a stye or a localised infection of the eyelid. It can affect the meibomian glands (internum) or eyelid hair follicles (externum).

K31 B: Pityriasis rosea

The Köbner phenomenon is the tendency for dermatological conditions to manifest themselves in areas of trauma, most typically seen with psoriasis but also in vitiligo, viral warts (especially plane warts) and lichen planus.

K32 E: Uveitis

A red eye is a medical emergency as the diseases responsible are able to lead to long-term damage and blindness. The main three to consider are closed angle glaucoma, acute conjunctivitis and uveitis. In this case the significant pain and photophobia suggest uveitis, which requires urgent ophthalmological assessment and steroid treatment.

QUESTIONS ON PAGES 66–67

K33   C: This condition is due to ankylosis

This patient is suffering from otosclerosis, which causes deafness due to fixation of the stapes footplate to the oval window. The hearing loss occurs during middle age and is typically exacerbated by pregnancy. Background noise masks the problem and actually improves the hearing. Audiometry shows a characteristic dip at 2 kHz. The condition can be inherited in an autosomal dominant manner, although roughly half of people affected have no family history. Females are affected twice as commonly as males, and most people who develop this condition suffer bilateral deafness. Tinnitus is also a common complaint. Those who undergo surgery for the condition risk deafness should the operation not work, with roughly 2%–5% of patients developing this complication.

K34   D: Churg–Strauss syndrome

Churg–Strauss is a rare vasculitis affecting small- and medium-sized vessels, especially within the lungs.

The presence of four or more of the criteria below is required for a diagnosis of the condition according to the American College of Rheumatology:

1. Asthma

2. Eosinophilia

3. Sinusitis

4. Lung infiltrates

5. Histological diagnosis of vasculitis with eosinophils

6. Mononeuritis multiplex or polyneuropathy

Treatment is with immunosuppression, commonly high-dose steroids, but occasionally cytotoxic drugs such as cyclophosphamide are needed.

K35 B: Atrial septal defect

Right bundle branch block and VSD cause wide splitting (but not classically fixed) while left bundle branch block and a patent ductus arteriosus cause reversed splitting of the second heart sound.

K36 E: Toilet Use

The areas assessed in the Barthel questionnaire are listed below, with a maximum score of 20 being attainable:

Bowels

Bladder

Grooming

Toilet use

Feeding

Transfer

Mobility

Dressing

Stairs

Bathing

QUESTIONS ON PAGE 69

K37   C: Metolazone is a powerful thiazide diuretic used in patients with severe and resistant heart failure

Loop diuretics exert their effects in the thick ascending limb of the loop of Henle via their action on Na/K/2Cl channels. Thiazide diuretics conversely affect the Na/Cl channel in the distal convoluted tubule. Metolazone is an example of an extremely potent thiazide diuretic commonly used synergistically with loop diuretics in resistant fluid overload, although great care has to be taken with monitoring electrolytes and renal function.

Amiloride is a weak potassium-sparing diuretic, commonly combined with thiazide diuretics, and inhibits sodium reabsorption in the collecting duct, thus limiting potassium excretion into urine.

Amiodarone has a wide range of side-effects and the main ones to monitor are thyroid function tests and liver function tests, although patients have to be counselled with regard to increased photosensitivity, lung fibrosis and corneal microdeposits.

Flecainide is a class I antiarrhythmic agent which has been shown to increase mortality in patients with significant coronary heart disease, left ventricular dysfunction or structural heart disease.

answers

K38   B: Sensory deprivation is a risk factor for the development of delirium

Delerium is a commonly encountered problem requiring admission among the elderly population and is frequently encountered on the ward, in both medical and surgical patients. The core features include:

1. Fluctuating course

2. Onset over hours to days

3. Clouding of consciousness

4. Impaired cognition

Confusion tends to get worse as the day progresses and leads to a reversal of the sleep cycle, leading to disturbances on the ward at night. Although sedatives should be avoided, occasionally it is in the patient's best interest to calm their behaviour slightly to prevent injuries and allow them to be looked after properly. Visual hallucinations occur commonly but care has to be taken to ascertain that they do not represent alcohol withdrawal hallucinations.

Patients with dementia are more likely to develop delirium and the two conditions often co-exist in hospitalised patients, but the majority of patients who have delirium do not have underlying dementia.

K39   E: The type V fracture is a crush fracture

A Salter–Harris fracture is one that occurs through an epiphyseal growth plate. As it is through a growth plate it can only occur in children before fusion of the epiphyses, with the type II fracture being the most common. Males are more frequently affected than females and careful reduction is needed to avoid problems with growth later. Greenstick fractures do not affect the growth plate and are therefore not included in the Salter–Harris classification.

QUESTIONS ON PAGE 70

K40 D: The tetanus vaccine is a toxin-based vaccine

Diphtheria, tetanus and polio vaccines are given a total of five times between birth and the age of 18.

The increase in measles seen is due the decreased uptake of the MMR vaccine, due to parental concerns with regard to the link between the MMR combined vaccine and autism. However all of the studies that have been conducted thus far, which are numerous and large, show no link between autism and the MMR vaccine.

Although being vaccinated is the most important factor in protecting individuals, herd immunity has a much bigger role in protecting the community. Herd immunity relies on a sufficiently large number of individuals being vaccinated so that in the event of an outbreak of an infection spread would be minimised and contained in the population, protecting both those immunised and unimmunised. When large numbers of individuals are unvaccinated, herd immunity no longer functions, thus putting a greater proportion of the population at risk.

The BCG vaccine is made from a live attenuated strain of *Mycobacterium bovis* and not *M. tuberculosis*.

Further information with regard to immunisations can be found at the extremely useful and easy-to-navigate NHS immunisations website (http://www.immunisation.nhs.uk) and the handy immunisation schedule available from the site is a useful quick reference guide.

K41 D: V/Q scan

This patient has dual pathology, with resolving pneumonia and a pulmonary embolus secondary to a deep vein thrombosis. The least useful investigation in this patient is a V/Q scan as the underlying pneumonia would make interpretation of a V/Q scan very difficult.

Pulse, blood pressure and ABG analysis are essential for ensuring the patient is stable and remains so. CT pulmonary angiography would be the best method to image the lungs in this case.

K42 A: Start antiviral therapy

The history in the scenario tries to trick you into thinking that there might be a cardiac cause, but the pain, tingling and the band-like erythema is more consistent with shingles, caused by herpes zoster. The best treatment is therefore antiviral therapy.

K43 B: Renal cell carcinoma

The constellation of signs and symptoms of an abdominal mass, haematuria and left varicocoele indicate an underlying renal cell carcinoma. A left varicocoele occurs in males due to compression or infiltration of the left testicular vein, which drains into the left renal vein. On the right-hand side the testicular vein joins the inferior vena cava.

Renal cell carcinoma has a well-known association with paraneoplastic syndromes, especially hypercalcaemia via ectopic parathyroid hormone and polycythaemia via excessive erythropoietin production.

Cannon-ball pulmonary metastases are a characteristic feature of renal cell carcinoma and testicular seminoma.

K44 C: Arrange for urgent catheterisation

This patient appears to have a palpable bladder and is therefore in urinary retention, thus accounting for the deterioration in his condition. The best diagnostic step is urinary catheterisation, as this will relieve the condition as well as diagnose it (by the large volume of urine released).

K45 D: Viral markers

The patient is suffering from oral and oesophageal candidiasis, with the most likely cause in this patient being underlying immunosuppression. Oesophageal candidiasis is an AIDS-defining condition, which necessitates careful counselling, risk factor analysis and testing for HIV.

K46   B: Parvovirus B19

This presentation, also known as 'fifth disease' and 'erythema infectiosum' is caused by parvovirus B19. Constitutional symptoms are usually mild and patients usually present with arthralgia. In patients with sickle cell disease and hereditary spherocytosis parvovirus B19 can lead to aplastic crises due to arrest of red cell production and if women are affected early in the course of a pregnancy there is a small but definite risk of miscarriage.

K47   E: The pregnancy test is usually positive 2 weeks after conception, not the last menstrual period

The pregnancy test is usually positive 2 weeks after conception and not the last menstrual period, although the missed period is the most common finding that alerts mothers to the pregnancy. All of the other statements are false. Haemoglobin levels fall due to dilution; ventilation and depth of breathing increase due to the increased demands of both mother and fetus. Cardiac output increases due to increased stroke volume and heart rate; and maternal cortisol output increases but levels stay fairly constant.

answers

K48 D: The majority of cold nodules seen on nuclear imaging of the thyroid are benign

Patients who are started on thyroxine replacement should have their thyroid function tests repeated every 6–8 weeks to assess the response and allow appropriate titration of the medication. In Graves' disease the stimulating antibodies against the TSH receptor are found on the follicular cells within the thyroid. Carbimazole and propylthiouracil exert their clinical effect by inhibiting the formation of thyroid hormones and not their release.

A nodule can be classified as cold or hot on the basis of nuclear medicine scans of the thyroid. Hot nodules are functioning and more than 95% of these are benign. Cold nodules represent a non-functioning area within the thyroid and although the majority of these are also benign, a closer eye is kept on them as they can indicate underlying malignancy. Solitary nodules are usually subjected to fine-needle aspiration and cytological analysis to delineate the underlying diagnosis clearly.

Papillary carcinoma of the thyroid is the commonest thyroid malignancy, followed by follicular thyroid cancer.

K49 D: Hyperparathyroidism increases the risk of developing the condition

The patient is suffering from chondrocalcinosis, also known as 'calcium pyrophosphate arthropathy'. Risk factors include age, dehydration, osteoarthritis and haemochromatosis. Acute attacks can resemble gout, except that the knee is most commonly affected. Osteoarthritis can be mistaken for the chronic form of the disease. Punched-out juxta-articular lesions occur more commonly with gout, as do needle-shaped, negatively birefringent crystals. Weakly positive birefringent rhomboidal crystals are more likely to be seen in chondrocalcinosis.

K50   C: The disease is associated with valvular heart disease

This history is consistent with ankylosing spondylitis, which is a seronegative arthropathy associated with HLA-B27. Males in their late teens are most commonly affected, suffering from back pain, morning stiffness and spinal ankylosis, which eventually leads to the characteristic question-mark posture. Patients with ankylosing spondylitis are at increased risk of valvular heart defects and secondary amyloidosis (AA amyloid) due to the chronic inflammation. All in all, patients are one and a half to two times more likely to die compared with a control population. Infliximab is a promising new agent that can be used in the treatment of ankylosing spondylitis.

K51   A: Fibroadenoma

Questions on breast pathology are a common part of all surgical exams and therefore an understanding of the common clinical pathologies, their mode of presentation and their management is important. In this patient, the young age and the description of the lump all point towards a diagnosis of fibroadenoma, although a red herring is the family history of breast cancer. Further management would include imaging, most likely to be ultrasound-based.

K52   E: Henoch–Schönlein purpura

Commonly said to be a systemic variant of IgA glomerulonephritis, the presentation is typical for HSP.

K53   A: Chronic lymphocytic leukaemia

The fullness in his abdomen indicates splenomegaly, which occurs in a quarter of patients with CLL. This leukaemia is seen most commonly in the elderly and has a variable course, often affecting the patient for a number of years but not causing significant distress. CLL is associated with autoimmune haemolysis caused by warm IgG antibodies, which causes red cell breakdown releasing free haemoglobin; this is scavenged by haptoglobin readily and thus accounts for a fall in haptoglobin levels. Other complications include aplastic anaemia and overwhelming sepsis.

K54   C: Request an urgent full blood count

This patient is a treated hyperthyroid patient and is therefore likely to be on carbimazole or propylthiouracil and so you have to be aware of the rare possibility of agranulocytosis and exclude this with a full blood count. Should the blood test show a low neutrophil count, urgent admission to hospital and treatment with broad-spectrum antibiotics is required, with cessation of carbimazole or propylthiouracil.

K55   B: Hereditary spherocytosis

Although adult polycystic kidney disease is autosomal dominant, the infantile form is autosomal recessive. In this case the answer is hereditary spherocytosis, which is typically inherited in an autosomal dominant fashion.

K56   C: Octreotide has a useful role in the above patient

The care of a dying patient requires a strong multidisciplinary team approach, including the patient's own team of doctors and nurses along with the palliative care services and hospices. Palliative care has a role not only in patients with cancer but also in any disease requiring support at the end of life, such as end-stage heart failure and COPD.

The Liverpool Care Pathway is a quality improvement framework which aims to improve the care of the dying patient in the hospital setting irrespective of the cause of the terminal condition.

Fluids are not routinely continued in the dying patient and medication is best given in a syringe driver to provide continuous analgesia with or without antiemetic cover, rather than the peak and trough therapy achieved with as-required medications, which should be used for breakthrough symptoms not controlled with the syringe driver.

In patients with bowel obstruction, as in this patient, prokinetic antiemetics are contraindicated and cyclizine and ondansetron would be better suited agents. Octreotide is useful in limiting gastric secretions.

K57   E: Adenosine

The patient has presented with a narrow-complex supraventricular tachycardia. The management involves oxygen administration followed by vagal manoeuvres such as the Valsalva manoeuvre, which terminates the attack in some patients.

Should this fail, adenosine can be attempted to block AV node conduction at an initial dose of 6 mg. The patient should be warned that they may feel 'impending doom', chest heaviness and flushing, but that these symptoms are short-lived.

Adenosine causes bronchospasm and is therefore contraindicated in patients with asthma, in whom verapamil or beta-blockers can be tried.

K58   B: Subthalamic nucleus

This famous symptom of flinging limb movements is caused by infarction of the contralateral subthalamic nucleus.

K59   D: Perianal haematoma

This is a clotted venous saccule, which can affect patients suffering from haemorrhoids. It is typically painful initially but responds to topical gels and does not cause pruritis ani.

K60   B: Diminished corneal reflex

A lesion of the cerebellopontine angle affects the fifth, seventh and eighth cranial nerves, classically followed by the development of ipsilateral cerebellar signs. The corneal reflex tests the trigeminal nerve sensory branch and its absence is a common finding in cerebellopontine angle tumours.

K61   A: Chronic arterial insufficiency is a likely underlying factor in this patient

This patient is suffering from an acute limb ischaemia as evident by the 6 'P's: Pain, Pallor, Paraesthesia, Pulseless, Paralysis and Perishing cold. A Fogarty catheter is used for surgical embolectomy and should be attempted if at all possible before a full open operation.

In patients with chronic arterial insufficiency a number of collaterals will have formed with time and they are thus less likely to develop acute ischaemia. An acute insult will therefore make their already poor circulation worse but the presence of collaterals should mean that they are relatively immune from developing the 6 'P's. Sympathectomy can be performed in chronic arterial insufficiency in an attempt to increase distal blood flow.

QUESTIONS ON PAGE 80

K62   A: The results are suggestive of viral meningitis

There are tables of the CSF appearances in normal subjects as well as in bacterial, tuberculous and viral meningitis in all medical textbooks.

Here the CSF glucose is greater than half of the blood glucose and the CSF protein is less than 1 g/l, which point towards a viral cause. Parasitic meningitis usually leads to low glucose and raised eosinophils in the CSF.

K63   D: Hypothyroidism

In hypothyroidism the MCV can be macrocytic while in all of the other cases the MCV is low or low–normal.

A short differential list for the causes of microcytic and macrocytic anaemia is always useful to have:

Microcytic:

> Iron deficiency
>
> Thalassaemia (usually a lower MCV than would be expected for the haemoglobin level)
>
> Sideroblastic anaemia, which when acquired has a number of causes
>
> Anaemia of chronic disease

Macrocytic:

> B12 and folate deficiency: nutritional as well as disease states such as pernicious anaemia and Crohn's disease with ileal involvement
>
> Alcohol
>
> Liver disease
>
> Hypothyroidism
>
> Reticulocytosis

K64   C: Cryoglobulinaemia

The key to solving the complex presentation in this patient is the past history of viral hepatitis, which in this case was likely to be hepatitis C. This has led to the formation of cryoglobulins; immunoglobulins which precipitate at lower temperatures. When this occurs the cryoglobulin complexes lead to vessel damage and ischaemia distal to the sites of complex deposition, commonly manifesting in Raynaud's phenomenon and discoloration of the nose and ears.

Cryoglobulinaemia is a multisystem disease leading to a number of symptoms, as described in the question: arthralgia, purpuric rash, Raynaud's phenomenon, glomerulonephritis and leg ulcers. In addition, confusion, neuropathy and manifestations of systemic vasculitis can occur.

The natural course can be variable, with a proportion of cases showing spontaneous remission while others require systemic immunosuppressive treatment.

K65   B: Hepatitis A

All viral hepatitis cases should be reported to a consultant in communicable disease.

It is wise to have some knowledge of what diseases need to be reported as it is a simple question to ask in exams. A full list of notifiable diseases is available from the Health Protection Agency: www.hpa.org.uk

K66   D: Diverticulitis

The age of the patient, along with the left-sided mass and tenderness, point towards a diagnosis of diverticulitis, which is becoming an increasingly common acute surgical presentation to hospitals. The patient is unwell and requires admission for intravenous fluids and antibiotics. A CT scan of the abdomen and pelvis will be useful to assess the extent of disease and evaluate the mass, which may represent a diverticular abscess.

QUESTIONS ON PAGES 82-83

K67 D: The patient should be given supportive care

The acid-base data shows an alkalosis, with a markedly decreased carbon dioxide suggesting respiratory alkalosis. Although she could be suffering from asthma the ability to complete sentences and the tingling in her limbs suggests hyperventilation and therefore supportive care and re-breathing into a paper bag is all that will be required.

K68 D: Normal-pressure hydrocephalus

The triad of dementia, incontinence and ataxia points towards this diagnosis.

K69 E: Alkalosis

Acidosis and not alkalosis is an urgent indication for dialysis.

K70 A: Squamous cell carcinoma

Raised calcium in this instance is most likely to be due to increased levels of parathyroid-related protein produced most commonly by squamous cell carcinoma, especially in the absence of identifiable metastatic disease.

K71 D: The pathogen is likely to be *Campylobacter jejuni*

All cases of food poisoning should be reported to the consultant in communicable disease. *Bacillus cereus* is responsible for fried rice food poisoning, due to rice that has been cooked then stored for a number of hours before being eaten. It causes symptoms within 2 hours of ingestion. *Salmonella* gastroenteritis also acts within 4–8 hours of ingestion. *Campylobacter jejuni* has a latent period of 2–5 days before symptoms become apparent.

The main treatment option in all cases of gastroenteritis is fluid rehydration, followed by antibiotics if required.

K72 E: Exercise tolerance test

This question raises the dilemma of whether this chest pain is cardiac in nature or secondary to a pulmonary embolus as there are features which favour both. The strong family history of cardiac disease, along with the central chest pain with radiation to the lower jaw is suspicious for cardiac disease while the stabbing pain, recent long-distance travel and the sister with a DVT point towards a PE.

However, taken together, the most likely diagnosis is exertional angina (the pain occurred while running for a bus) and the negative blood test at 12 hours suggests this is troponin-negative chest pain.

The most appropriate investigation is an exercise tolerance test, which will allow us to risk-stratify the patient. Ischaemic changes on the ECG can then be investigated further with a coronary angiogram to investigate for significant coronary stenosis and appropriate management can be planned.

K73 C: Cystic hygroma

This is the typical appearance of a dilated lymphatic system in the neck. Knowledge of neck lumps is vital as they are commonly tested: it is best to divide them into which triangle of the neck they occur in.

K74 B: Pain, jaundice and fever

Charcot's triad for ascending cholangitis is pain, jaundice and fever. This is a commonly occurring theme in single best answer questions and extended matching questions.

The key differentials are biliary colic and acute cholecystitis.

K75   B: 45%

This question demands you know about Wallace's rule of nines, which is used in assessing the percentage of body surface affected by burns:

Front of body	18%
Back of body	18%
Left arm	9% (includes 1% for the hand)
Right arm	9% (includes 1% for the hand)
Left leg	18% (front 9%, back 9%)
Right leg	18% (front 9%, back 9%)
Head and neck	9%
Genital area	1%

K76   C: Soft second heart sound

In aortic stenosis the intensity and loudness of the murmur is not a good guide to severity because the murmur can become fairly quiet with decreasing cardiac output. A collapsing pulse would be expected in aortic regurgitation and not in aortic stenosis, where a slow-rising pulse is characteristically palpable.

Aortic stenosis can be graded according to the valve area, which is normally 3−4 cm²:

Mild	> 1.5 cm²
Moderate	1.0−1.05 cm²
Severe	< 1 cm²

A soft second heart sound implies severe aortic stenosis and is a useful clinical observation to make in patients with an ejection systolic murmur.

K77   C: Haloperidol

The patient has developed neuroleptic malignant syndrome as a result of the haloperidol he was given for his behavioural difficulties. Treatment of neuroleptic malignant syndrome includes withdrawing the precipitant and supportive care. Dantrolene and full anaesthesia can also be used.

K78   D: Supportive management

This patient has suffered a subarachnoid haemorrhage (SAH) and supportive management is all that is indicated at present. Although CT scanning is the first-line imaging modality it can miss a small percentage of SAH, in which case lumbar puncture should be performed at least 6–12 hours after onset of the headache to allow for bilirubin to be detected in the CSF, which is only produced in vivo as opposed to oxyhaemaglobin which is also present in a traumatic tap.

A useful resource is:

Al-Shahi R et al. Subarachnoid haemorrhage. *BMJ* 2006; 333: 235–40.

K79   B: Transitional cell carcinoma

Painless haematuria should always raise a suspicion of transitional cell carcinoma until proved otherwise.

K80   A: Oligohydramnios

This patient with a large-for-date uterus and hyperemesis gravidarum is likely to have been carrying twins, a fact diagnosed on ultrasound. Twin pregnancies are at greater risk of nearly all the complications faced by a single pregnancy except for oligohydramnios.

K81   D: The patient is suffering from paraphimosis

When undertaking male catheterisation it is important to replace the foreskin after completion of the procedure. If this is not carried out paraphimosis can occur, which is where the retracted foreskin cannot be pulled back over the corona of the penis.

K82   C: Posterior dislocation of the hip

The description given in the case applies only to a posterior dislocation of the hip. A fractured neck of femur would lead to a shortened and externally rotated limb.

K83   A: Patients with the condition are at increased risk of developing coronary heart disease

A swan-neck deformity is due to hyperextension at the proximal interphalangeal (PIP) joint and flexion at the distal interphalangeal (DIP) joint. A boutonnière deformity is due to flexion at the PIP and extension at the DIP joints. Felty syndrome is the association of rheumatoid arthritis, splenomegaly and neutropenia. HLA-DR4 is one of the commonest HLA types associated with rheumatoid arthritis and its incidence is much higher in those affected by Felty syndrome.

K84   B: L5

Knowledge of dermatomes and myotomes is essential for undertaking an accurate neurological examination.

K85   E: 11

Examiners can very easily ask questions based on the Glasgow coma scale:

Eyes:

4 – Spontaneously open

3 – Open to speech

2 – Open to pain

1 – No opening

Voice:

5 – Normal orientated speech

4 – Confused speech

3 – Random or inappropriate words

2 – Sounds not words

1 – No vocalisation

Motor:

6 – Spontaneous movements/obeying commands

5 – Localises pain

4 – Withdraws from pain

3 – Flexor response

2 – Extensor response

1 – No motor response to pain

5 + 4 + 2 = GCS of 11

K86   A: Neck X-ray

Patients with rheumatoid arthritis can have involvement of the cervical spine, causing an increased risk of subluxation and significant injury while positioning a patient's head for intubation and anaesthesia. A vital examination in a patient with a history of rheumatoid arthritis is a neck X-ray to assess the degree of damage and allow anaesthetists to take the above into consideration.

QUESTIONS ON PAGE 93

K87   D: Patients suffering from borderline personality disorder can be sectioned for assessment and treatment

Section 2 allows detention for assessment (and/or treatment) of a patient with a suspected mental disorder against their will for a maximum of 28 days.

Section 3 allows detention and treatment of a patient for a psychiatric disorder against their will for a maximum of 6 months.

Section 4 allows a patient to be brought into hospital in an emergency for further assessment. It should be rapidly changed to a Section 2 or 3 as appropriate.

Section 136 allows police officers to bring an individual from a public area to medical attention and to a place of safetty, should the police officers feel that the individual is suffering from a mental illness.

Section 5(4) allows a nurse and Section 5(2) allows a doctor to detain a patient who they feel is suffering a psychiatric illness until they are formally assessed by the psychiatric team.

The Emergency Department does not count as a hospital ward.

K88   A: Xeroderma pigmentosa

Xeroderma pigmentosa is autosomal recessive whereas the others are autosomal dominant.

K89   B: Magnesium-containing antacids can relieve constipation

Fybogel is a bulking agent which should be used with plenty of fluids. Co-danthramer is a stimulant laxative used exclusively in the terminally ill because of its carcinogenic and genotoxic side-effects. Lactulose is an osmotic laxative that can take 2 days to work.

Magnesium in certain antacids has a laxative effect on the colon while antacids which contain aluminium cause constipation. Hypokalaemia is a much greater risk than hyperkalaemia with excessive use of laxatives.

K90   E: Levels of a subunit of the MHC class I unit provides useful prognostic information

This patient has underlying multiple myeloma (MM) accounting for the presentation described. Alkaline phosphatase is usually within normal limits unless a fracture has occurred and punched-out lesions are common with MM. Urine electrophoresis detects immunoglobulin light chains, which are produced in excess and known as 'Bence Jones' proteins.

Beta-2-microglobulin is a subunit of the MHC class I molecule and provides useful prognostic information in MM.

K91   D: Spirometry

This patient is likely to have Guillain–Barré syndrome, which is an acute inflammatory demyelinating polyradiculopathy that leads to progressive weakness. It has a progressive course and can be very severe, potentially requiring mechanical ventilation if the respiratory muscles are severely affected. To monitor this the most useful investigation is spirometry to assess the forced vital capacity, with any downward trend an indication for early intervention.

Due to prolonged immobility and a gradual recovery, prophylactic heparin is indicated. Treatment includes supportive care, intravenous immunoglobulins and plasma exchange. Although steroids were used previously current data show no benefit from their use.

K92   C: Barium swallow

Given the lack of history for gastro-oesophageal reflux disease, gastric/duodenal ulcers or sinister pathology, a barium swallow would be the most useful method to assess this patient.

K93   A: Hodgkin's lymphoma

The Reed–Sternberg cell is characteristically associated with Hodgkin's lymphoma. It is a large multinucleated cell, derived from B lymphocytes, and has highly eosinophilic inclusion bodies.

K94   C: SHOT

Serious Hazards Of Transfusion is a monitoring scheme to analyse transfusion-related errors and adverse outcomes.

K95   A: Thyroid-stimulating hormone

From the list given, TSH is the most useful investigation as it is nearly always reduced in hyperthyroidism (except in the exceedingly rare case of a TSH-secreting tumour).

K96   E: *Staphylococcus aureus*

Influenza can be complicated by pneumonia, as has occurred in this patient. The commonest organism reported is *Staphylococcus aureus* and the bilateral upper lobe involvement with cavitation is in keeping with this.

K97   B: Teaching undergraduate medical students to further improve medical knowledge

Clinical governance is a wide-ranging concept that aims to continually improve clinical services through regular audits, use of evidence-based medicine, risk reduction and outcome reviews. Teaching medical students does not form part of clinical governance.

K98   C: Gastro-oesophageal reflux disease

The most common cause of an oesophageal stricture is acid reflux disease. All of the others can lead to stricture formation but are much rarer.

K99   B: Ekbom syndrome

Also known as 'restless leg syndrome', the presentation described is characteristic.

Akathisia is an inability to get comfortable and at rest, no matter which position a patient adopts and is a side-effect of certain neuroleptics.

K100   E: Rosiglitazone

This patient presents in heart failure due to a change in her diabetic medication. The most likely cause is the introduction of a glitazone, which, although useful in managing diabetes, has the side-effect of fluid retention.

K101   C: Dilated cardiomyopathy

This patient presents in severe heart failure with the most likely diagnosis being alcohol-related dilated cardiomyopathy, which can be inferred from the raised MCV.

K102   D: Poxvirus

This patient is suffering from molluscum contagiosum caused by the poxvirus.

answers

K103   C: GTN Infusion

This gentleman has been treated for pulmonary oedema in the Emergency Department and brought to the ward. Unfortunately he has gone back into pulmonary oedema on the ward, which should be treated by sitting the patient upright, administering morphine, an antiemetic and intravenous furosemide. If this is not satisfactory a GTN infusion should be started, which should be slowly increased and titrated to ensure the blood flow does drop precipitously.

After this, continuous positive airway pressure (CPAP) ventilation can be considered, by which time the F1 should have called for experienced help and organised initial investigations such as blood tests, ABG, chest X-ray and especially ECG (in view of the irregular pulse).

Acute pulmonary oedema is a common emergency faced on the wards and a basic knowledge is therefore vital.

K104   E: Needle aspiration in 2nd intercostal space, mid-clavicular line

This patient is likely to have a tension pneumothorax, evidenced by the deviated trachea, respiratory distress and resonant percussion note, and urgent treatment is therefore required.

K105   E: Diabetes Insipidus

The water deprivation test is classically used in the diagnosis of diabetes insipidus. Water is withheld so that the plasma osmolality rises to > 290 mosmol/kg, a concentration sufficient to stimulate ADH release. The normal physiological response is for urine to be concentrated > 600 mosmol/kg but in diabetes insipidus it remains dilute at < 350 mosmol/kg. Desmopressin can then given to elucidate whether it is cranial (lack of ADH release) or nephrogenic (lack of response to ADH) diabetes insipidus.

answers

K106   C: Anti-HBs antibody

Hepatitis B surface antigen is present in an acute infection, with levels becoming undetectable after a few months. If hepatitis B surface antigen persists it signifies a chronic infection.

Hepatitis B e antigen implies increased infectivity until anti-HBe antibodies are made, which indicate decreasing infectivity.

Anti-HBc is the first antibody to be produced and is therefore IgM, with levels persisting for years, and can indicate previous exposure to hepatitis B.

Anti-HBs antibodies indicate immunity and are the antibodies routinely tested in healthcare workers to ensure hepatitis B vaccinations have triggered a sufficient immunological reaction.

K107   A: Discharge

This patient has a relatively small (< 2 cm) primary pneumothorax and current treatment guidelines recommend that patients such as this can be discharged from the Emergency Department without active therapy. However, he should be reviewed in 2 weeks' time in a chest or general medicine clinic with a repeat chest X-ray.

The following guidelines, developed by the British Thoracic Society are a useful resource:

Henry M et al. British Thoracic Society Guidelines for the management of spontaneous pneumothorax. *Thorax* 2003; 58, Supplement 2: 39–52.

K108   D: ECG

This patient has most likely taken an overdose of tricyclic antidepressant (TCA) medications, accounting for the significant anticholinergic side-effects seen. TCA overdose can cause fatal cardiac arrhythmias in addition to coma and hypothermia. An ECG should be undertaken in the first instance, with a prolonged QRS complex suggestive of a significant overdose.

K109 D: Vasculitis

This patient is suffering from Wegener's granulomatosis, a vasculitis which affects the upper and lower respiratory tract and kidneys. It is a systemic small-vessel vasculitis which is classically SP3 anti-neutrophil cytoplasmic antibody (c-ANCA) positive.

K110 D: Surgical referral

The underlying diagnosis in this patient is nasal polyps, which are benign soft-tissue growths occurring on the sinus mucosa. They are thought to result from chronic irritation secondary to allergic rhinitis, sinusitis or inflammation and in young children are often associated with cystic fibrosis.

His nasal polyps are significant given that they have started to affect his smell and sleep and therefore surgical referral is warranted. Further investigations include allergy testing, given his allergic asthma, to allow him to exclude any precipitants from his environment, as well as a fibreoptic nasal endoscopy in an ENT clinic, along with a CT or MRI scan.

Various treatments are available, including oral or intranasal steroid sprays, anti-inflammatory medications and leukotriene antagonists. Surgical polypectomy is a useful option in patients with large or multiple polyps.

K111 A: Small-bowel biopsy

This patient is suffering from Whipple's disease, which is diagnosed using small-bowel biopsy and staining to show PAS-positive macrophages. The organism responsible is *Tropheryma whipplei,* which can be effectively treated with antibiotics.

K112   E: Patient-controlled analgesia

Pain relief is a vital part of the management of the postsurgical patient. Patient-controlled analgesia (PCA) is an extremely useful method to control pain as it is patient-operated and can deliver pain relief when needed or when it will be expected without having repeatedly to ask nurses or doctors for tablets.

K113   A: Hyperkalaemia

The side-effects of steroids should be memorised as they are used extensively and questions based on their side-effects also occur frequently.

Side effects include:

Cardiovascular: hypertension

Fluid balance: sodium and water retention, hypokalaemia

Endocrine: diabetes, osteoporosis, and Cushing syndrome – thin skin, change of body fat stores, easy bruising and adrenal suppression

Gastrointestinal: peptic ulceration

Psychiatric: euphoria/depression/altered mental state

Miscellaneous: avascular necrosis of the femoral head, increased susceptibility to infections

British National Formulary (BNF) 50, September 2005.

K114   C: Dosage in words

All prescriptions should be filled out in the correct manner with all of the appropriate information. Due to the nature of controlled drugs, further security measures are needed, but writing the dosage in words does not form part of that.

The number of tablets or amount of solution to be prescribed has to be written in figures and words.

K115   B: Alopecia areata

The tapering of hairs proximally, also known as 'exclamation mark' hair is a classic finding in alopecia areata. Pitting of the nails is not exclusively seen in psoriasis.

K116   D: Sigmoidoscopy

In an outpatient clinic it would be advisable first to undertake a digital rectal examination followed by rigid sigmoidoscopy, which allows visualisation of the anorectal region.

K117   D: Furosemide

Furosemide in high doses is ototoxic and patients requiring significant quantities of furosemide to offload fluid are at high risk.

K118   B: Acute onset

Good and poor prognostic features in schizophrenia:

Good Prognosis	Poor prognosis
Satisfactory social relationships	Early onset
Satisfactory academic performance	Gradual onset
Satisfactory work performance	No precipitant
Late onset	Negative symptoms
Acute onset	Abnormal CT scan
Psychological precipitant	Little response to medication
Positive symptoms	Learning difficulties
Normal CT scan	
Good response to medication	

K119   A: Iatrogenic

A raised JVP with a normal waveform is a sign of high right atrial pressure and is commonly due to fluid overload by overzealous fluid replacement.

In superior vena cava obstruction there is a raised JVP with absent pulsation, along with the other features of SVC obstruction, namely oedematous and erythematous face and neck. Pulmonary stenosis leads to a large 'a' wave whereas complete heart block leads to cannon 'a' waves in which the right atrium contracts against a closed tricuspid valve.

In constrictive pericarditis there is a paradoxical rise in the JVP on inspiration (Kussmaul's sign).

K120   A: Hypertension

Hypertension is the leading cause of atrial fibrillation in the community because of the high prevalence of the condition (even though any single hypertensive patient is at a low risk of developing AF).

K121   B: Flumazenil

The patient is likely to have been given too much midazolam and the antidote in the acute setting is flumazenil. Patients who take benzodiazepines chronically and also take an overdose should not be given flumazenil routinely as they can suffer a marked withdrawal reaction.

K122   C: Post-streptococcal glomerulonephritis

Berger's disease or IgA nephropathy is a common form of glomerulonephritis which affects males more than females and presents with recurrent macroscopic haematuria, usually triggered by infections in children and young adults.

Buerger's disease affects young male smokers and is also known as 'thromboangiitis obliterans'. It is a result of non-atherosclerotic arterial compromise, leading to rest pain, arterial ulcers and gangrene. Abstaining from tobacco consumption is the main form of treatment.

Post-streptococcal glomerulonephritis (PSGN) is an acute glomerulonephritis that can occur after throat or skin infection with certain strains of *Streptococcus*, almost always group A. It leads to haematuria, proteinuria, oedema, hypertension and acute renal failure.

In Berger's disease haematuria and glomerulonephritis occur 1–2 days after an infection while PSGN usually presents 2 weeks after infection.

K123   D: Tazocin and gentamicin intravenously

This patient has presented with neutropenic sepsis, as defined by the low neutrophil count. The patient should have multiple cultures taken, including blood, urine, sputum and faeces, in order to find the responsible pathogen (although in reality the pathogen responsible is identified in fewer than 50% of cases).

Suitable and prompt antibiotic therapy is a definite requirement and from the list given Tazocin and gentamicin are the two antibiotics that are usually given to cover neutropenic sepsis.

answers

K124   C: A peripheral lesion of the trigeminal nerve leads to deviation of the jaw towards the side of the lesion

A lesion in the hypoglossal or trigeminal nerve causes the tongue or jaw to deviate towards the side of the lesion respectively. A lesion in the vagus nerve causes the palate to deviate to the normal side.

Gradenigo syndrome is the triad of otorrhoea, retro-orbital pain and sixth nerve palsy and is a complication of otitis media and mastoiditis of the petrous temporal bone.

The facial nerve provides parasympathetic fibres to the salivary glands.

K125   B: Cirrhosis

The patient has a pleural effusion which was tapped.

Pneumonia, pancreatitis, SLE and mesothelioma all lead to an exudate whereas cirrhosis leads to a transudate.

Light's criteria help you to differentiate between a transudate and an exudate when faced with a pleural effusion. If one or more of the following is satisfied, the pleural fluid is likely to be an exudate:

- Pleural fluid protein/serum protein > 0.5

- Pleural fluid lactate dehydrogenase (LDH)/serum LDH > 0.6

- Pleural fluid LDH more than two-thirds above the upper limit of normal for serum LDH

K126   D: Ciprofloxacin

Augmentin is a combination of amoxicillin and clavulanic acid and Tazocin contains piperacillin and tazobactam. Ceftriaxone and cefuroxime are both cephalosporins and 5% to 10% of patients allergic to penicillins are also allergic to cephalosporins and caution is therefore advised. The safest antibiotic from the above list is therefore ciprofloxacin.

K127   C: Ankylosis

Ankylosis occurs in ankylosing spondylitis and not osteoarthritis. All of the others are classic features of osteoarthritis.

K128   B: Laxative abuse

Melanosis coli is a dark-brown/black appearance of the colonic mucosa due to pigment-filled macrophages that occurs with overuse of laxatives, especially senna.

K129   E: Propylthiouracil

The patient has symptoms of hyperthyroidism, secondary to Graves' disease, given the characteristic eye signs. Treatment is required in pregnancy as uncontrolled hyperthyroidism can lead to adverse outcomes for both the fetus and mother.

Radioactive iodine is contraindicated in pregnancy due to irradiation of the fetal thyroid and surgery should be used as a last resort. The most appropriate therapy is therefore propylthiouracil, which is the anti-thyroid medication of choice during pregnancy.

A useful review: Marx H et al. Hyperthyroidism and pregnancy. *BMJ* 2008; 336: 663–7.

K 130 C: Identify and name two objects

The Mini Mental State Examination:

– Day, date, month, year, season	5
– Country, town, street, building, floor	5
– Repeat and memorise three objects	3
– Serial sevens or WORLD backwards	5
– Recall three objects (from above)	3
– Follow a three-step command	3
– Name two objects after being shown them	2
– Read and follow the sentence 'Close your eyes'	1
– Write a sentence of your choosing	1
– Repeat 'No ifs, ands or buts'	1
– Copy two intersecting pentagons	1
Total	30

Abbreviated Mental Test Score:

– Memorise an address and recall it later	1
– Age	1
– Time	1
– Year	1
– Date of birth	1
– Name of hospital	1
– Name two people (doctor and nurse)	1
– Date of World War I or World War II	1
– Current monarch	1
– Count from 20 to 1 backwards	1
Total	10

QUESTION ON PAGE 113

K131   B: Gilbert syndrome and Crigler–Najjar syndrome lead to jaundice through defects in the same enzyme

Jaundice is clinically detectable with bilirubin concentrations of 35–40 μmol/l, an AST:ALT ratio of 2:1 is highly suggestive of alcoholic liver disease and bilirubin is converted to urobilinogen in the gut by bacteria.

Anti-mitochondrial antibodies are also found in chronic active hepatitis and idiopathic cirrhosis and are not specific to primary biliary cirrhosis.

Gilbert syndrome and Crigler–Najjar syndrome lead to jaundice through a defect in UDP-glucuronosyltransferase. In the former there is decreased activity of the enzyme while in the latter there is complete lack of the enzyme.

K132   A: Confusion

The severity of pneumonia can be measured by assessing the **CURB-65 score**, with two or more features suggestive of a severe pneumonia

– **C**onfusion

– **U**rea > 7 mmol/l

– **R**espiratory rate > 30/minute

– **B**lood pressure < 90 mmHg systolic (< 60 mmHg diastolic)

– **65** years or older

As the score gets higher the corresponding risk of death also rises, with a risk of less than 5% with a score of 0–1 and reaching 50% for a score of between 4 and 5.

answers

K133 A: The disease responds to prednisolone treatment

This patient has polymyalgia rheumatica, an inflammatory condition which requires steroid treatment, with most cases responding well to steroids. It usually affects females and is usually seen after the age of 50. Morning stiffness is a common finding and is in keeping with the above diagnosis. The ESR is typically raised significantly and you should always consider the complication of giant-cell arteritis, which is associated with this condition.

K134 E: Urine test

The triad of headaches associated with anxiety and hypertension makes a phaeochromocytoma a strong possibility in this patient. A 24-hour urine collection and analysis for metanephrines should be undertaken.

K135 C: Oral erythropoietin

Erythropoietin is a hormone delivered to patients by subcutaneous or intravenous injection and is not taken orally.

K136 D: Patients who still remain breathless after maximal medical therapy should be considered for surgery

The diagnosis and management of both exacerbations of COPD and stable COPD is a common exam topic and vital for life on the wards, where a large number of patients will have COPD.

Tiotropium is a long-acting anticholinergic and is not related to theophylline.

Inhaled corticosteroids should be started when the FEV_1 is less than 50% of that predicted. Night-time waking along with large improvements in FEV_1 and FEV_1/FVC with steroids is more in keeping with asthma than with COPD. Patients with COPD also have chronic irreversible lung damage and therefore even with maximal medical therapy we would not expect the FEV_1 and FEV_1/FVC to return to normal.

In patients with breathlessness and limitation of their daily activities even with maximal medical therapy and pulmonary rehabilitation, a number of forms of surgical treatments are available, including bullectomy, lung volume reduction surgery and, in severe cases, lung transplantation.

Smoking cessation is very important in the management of COPD and should be encouraged whenever possible.

A useful resource is the British Thoracic Society Guidelines on the diagnosis and management of COPD, which form the basis of most exam questions: http://www.brit-thoracic.org.uk/

K137 E: Small kidneys

Although anaemia develops in chronic renal failure secondary to a deficiency in erythropoietin, anaemia can also develop for a number of other reasons. High urea levels lead to hypertension and gastritis but gastritis can also occur independently of any kidney problem. Hyperkalaemia occurs in both acute and chronic renal failure and the creatinine levels bear no relation to the chronicity of the renal pathology.

Bilateral shrunken kidneys, typically detected on ultrasound examination, are therefore most suggestive of chronic renal failure.

K138 E: Rigidity is worsened with voluntary movement in the contralateral limb

Parkinson's disease is more common in males than in females. The presence of dementia at the time of diagnosis suggests an alternative diagnosis. Levodopa is combined with dopa-decarboxylase inhibitors to increase the availability of levodopa to the brain and not COMT inhibitors (although they can also be used in the treatment of Parkinson's disease).

K139 D: Patients with primary biliary cirrhosis typically have raised serum cholesterol levels

The leading cause of cirrhosis worldwide is chronic viral infections, followed closely by alcohol. In Budd–Chiari syndrome there is obstruction of the hepatic vein, while schistosomiasis results in intrahepatic portal hypertension. Non-alcoholic steatohepatitis is a more severe form of non-alcoholic fatty liver disease and is thought to be a significant cause of cirrhosis.

K140 A: Fibrates are agonist of the PPAR-α receptor and raise HDL cholesterol levels

Ezetimibe lowers serum cholesterol by inhibiting the intestinal absorption of cholesterol.

Familial hypercholesterolaemia (FH) is autosomal dominant in its inheritance and the heterozygous form affects approximately 1 in 500 people, the principal defect being with the LDL receptor.

The incidence of hypercholesterolaemia is not normally distributed but is bimodal, one peak occurring in young children and adults affected by FH and another larger peak occurring in adults with polygenic and lifestyle-related hypercholesterolaemia.

The commonest cause of hypercholesterolaemia is in fact polygenic hypercholesterolaemia, which is a susceptible genotype combined with adverse lifestyle factors.

Fibrates are agonists of the PPAR-α receptor (peroxisome proliferator-activated receptor) and exert their beneficial effects by raising levels of HDL cholesterol (the good cholesterol) and decreasing triglyceride levels.

K141   B: Measure serum ferritin

Although the most common site of blood loss in an elderly patient with microcytic anaemia is the gastrointestinal tract, it is wise to measure serum ferritin to ensure that the microcytic anaemia is due to iron deficiency.

K142   B: Amiodarone

Amiodarone is a medication used to treat a range of arrhythmias but which has a number of significant side-effects, including hypo- or hyperthyroidism, corneal microdeposits, pulmonary fibrosis, and skin discoloration due to phototoxicity.

He is unlikely to be on beta-blockers because of his asthma and the clue in the question is that he has poorly controlled atrial fibrillation.

K143   D: Colchicine

This patient is likely to be suffering from gout, which has been brought about by the treatment of his heart failure with diuretics. The key diagnosis to exclude is septic arthritis, although there is no evidence of this in the scenario.

Treatment of an acute attack of gout includes pain relief and rehydration (although cautiously in view of his heart failure). NSAIDs are frequently used but are contraindicated in this patient as they lead to fluid retention and would exacerbate his heart failure. Aspirin can aggravate gout and allopurinol in the acute setting will make gout worse.

Colchicine is therefore the most suitable treatment.

K144   D: Hypotension

In raised intracranial pressure bradycardia is accompanied by hypertension and a sixth nerve lesion is a false localising sign.

answers

K145   D: Aminophylline

Activated charcoal should be to given in aminophylline overdoses to prevent absorption and increase elimination. It is of no benefit in overdoses with the other agents.

K146   C: Anti-glomerular basement membrane antibodies

This patient is suffering from Goodpasture's disease, a type II hypersensitivity reaction in which the antibodies target the glomerular basement membrane and lungs, leading to haemoptysis and renal failure.

K147   C: Diabetic ketoacidosis is an important differential diagnosis

This patient presents with the common surgical presentation of appendicitis. Mortality is highest in the elderly, especially those over the age of 70, because of atypical and delayed presentation. Rovsig's sign is pain in the right iliac fossa on palpation of the left iliac fossa. Leukocytosis, not lymphocytosis, is present in 80% to 90% of patients. Appendicitis is the commonest non-obstetric surgical emergency in pregnancy.

Abdominal pain has numerous differentials, both surgical and medical, with diabetic ketoacidosis being an important one that is frequently forgotten.

K148   D: Behçet's disease

Behçet's disease is a rare but characteristic disease usually affecting men from around the Mediterranean basin. The classic features of Behçet's include:

- Recurrent oral aphthous ulceration

- A range of skin lesions, including erythema nodosum

- Eye lesions, including uveitis and iritis

- Genital ulceration

- Arthritis

- Epididymitis

- Central nervous system disturbances

- Pathergy: erythematous papule at the site of a needle puncture mark after 24–48 hours

K149   C: Dexamethasone suppression test

This patient has presented with hyponatraemia, which has a number of causes. Plasma lipids and glucose measurement excludes pseudo-hyponatraemia. Hyponatraemia can also be caused by SIADH, in which urine sodium and osmolality would be useful to exclude or diagnose this.

The dexamethasone suppression test is used in the diagnosis of Cushing's disease, in which patients would typically retain sodium and thus be hypernatraemic.

K150   A: Lugol's iodine

Thyrotoxic crisis is an endocrine emergency and should be treated with propylthiouracil or carbimazole (the former also inhibits peripheral conversion), steroids, beta-blockers and fluids.

Lugol's iodine should not be used acutely as it can lead to further thyroid hormone release but it can be used a few hours after anti-thyroid medication to help inhibit thyroid function.

K151   C: Cystic fibrosis

The FEV_1/FVC is 1.75/2 = 88%, which indicates a restrictive lung defect. Causes can be musculoskeletal or intrapulmonary, including many of the diseases listed, but not cystic fibrosis, which causes an obstructive defect.

K152   C: Sitting the patient upright is contraindicated

This patient has inadvertently received spinal anaesthesia instead of epidural anaesthesia and if not corrected this can lead to respiratory arrest. It is vital to alert the on-call anaesthetist urgently and stop the infusion of bupivacaine.

Sitting the patient upright will cause a catastrophic drop in blood pressure as the local anaesthetic has blocked the sympathetic outflow and the patient has no means by which to raise their blood pressure or heart rate.

K153   D: Urine test

This patient has features suggestive of Wilson's disease, an autosomal recessive condition in which total body copper stores are higher than usual, leading to copper deposition in organs such as the liver and basal ganglia, leading to cirrhosis and movement disorders. A 24-hour urine collection shows increased urinary copper and is a better test than serum copper levels.

K154   B: Incision and drainage of the abscess would be recommended in this patient

This patient has a pilonidal sinus that has become infected and now presents with an abscess, thus requiring surgical debridement. Women are less commonly affected than men, but those who are usually develop the condition earlier because of earlier hormonal changes. Pilonidal sinus disease is more common in whites than in Africans and Asians and, as would be expected, obesity is a risk factor. Meticulous hygiene and close shaving of the affected area can in some cases have a dramatic effect in controlling the disease.

K155   C: Bronchopneumonia

Death is rarely caused by Parkinson's disease itself, with most patients succumbing to a chest infection.

K156   C: Blood glucose measurement

This patient has a BMI of $150/1.75^2 = 49$ kg/m^2. The rash is most likely to be intertrigo with secondary bacterial infection.

The most useful investigation in this patient is blood glucose measurement as she is likely to have frank diabetes as well as a number of associated medical problems.

K157   A: A respiratory alkalosis would be in keeping with this overdose

Aspirin or salicylate overdose leads to a respiratory alkalosis initially because of direct stimulation of the respiratory centre before the development of a metabolic acidosis. Unlike paracetamol overdose, patients who take a large overdose of aspirin typically present with nausea, vomiting, tinnitus, sweating and general malaise within the first 24 hours.

In all cases of overdose a number of medications might have been taken and so it is routine to also send for paracetamol levels to be analysed.

Plasma concentrations of salicylates are helpful:

- < 300 mg/l is therapeutic

- 500–750 mg/l is a moderate overdose

- > 750 mg/l is a severe overdose – with acute renal failure being a real danger in these patients

K158   B: Significant drop in jugular venous pressure on inspiration

This patient has a cardiac tamponade and we would expect Beck's triad of muffled heart sounds, falling blood pressure and tachycardia to be present. The JVP would also be raised and would rise on inspiration (Kussmaul's sign) rather than fall.

K159   E: *Clostridium perfringens*

The sign of crepitations on palpation is highly suggestive of gas gangrene, caused by the above organism. It is a very severe infection leading to rapid muscle necrosis, gas production and sepsis, which occurs once the organism encounters favourable anaerobic conditions.

Definitive treatment is excision of dead and decaying muscle with wide excision margins and prompt antibiotics.

K160   C: Scabies

The description given is classic for scabies. In older children and adults the face is typically not involved but in infants and young children it can be affected.

K161   D: Patients should have a PaO$_2$ less than 7.3 kPa to be suitable for LTOT

Long-term oxygen therapy has been shown to substantially decrease mortality in those who qualify for it if used for more than 15 hours a day. Patients should therefore be advised to keep oxygen on for more than 15 hours, not 5 hours. Mortality decreases by 50% over the space of a few years. When assessing patients for LTOT, two arterial blood gas readings should be taken when the patient is stable. They should be undertaken with the patient breathing room air and a few weeks apart. Patients who have polycythaemia or secondary complications such as cor pulmonale are eligible for LTOT with a PaO$_2$ of < 8 kPa.

K162 B: Scalp tenderness

Scalp tenderness is not a classic feature of migraine and points more towards a diagnosis of giant-cell arteritis. All of the other features can occur in a migraine.

K163 A: Serum free light chains

The diagnosis is likely to be multiple myeloma and therefore the most useful investigation is assessment for serum free light chains.

K164 A: Age of 40

Red flags for back pain include altered bowel motions, bilateral sciatica, sleep disturbance with no rest at night, in addition to options B and E. Discitis should be an important consideration in people with PUO and back pain because this can progress to complete destruction of the vertebrae, leading to spinal cord compression, if not detected and treated in time.

An age of less than 20 or greater than 60 is significant for sinister pathology in patients presenting with acute-onset or severe back pain.

K165 A: The ambulance should take the patient to the tertiary referral centre for primary percutaneous coronary intervention

Numerous trials have compared thrombolysis with percutaneous coronary intervention (PCI), with the findings suggesting primary percutaneous coronary intervention has better outcomes over thrombolysis even if patients have to be transferred to a tertiary referral centre in order for treatment to be delivered. This is provided that the time for transfer is not excessive and the patient is stable for transfer.

Many regions now instruct paramedics to take all STEMI patients straight to a predetermined tertiary referral centre for coronary angiography and/or balloon angioplasty and/or stent insertion.

If PCI is unavailable thrombolysis should be undertaken as soon as possible – 'time is muscle'.

K166   B: Stool consistency

Features of a severe attack of ulcerative colitis can be remembered using the following memory aid – **Bloody FEAST**:

Bloody	Haemoglobin < 10.5 g/dl
F	Fever
E	Raised ESR
A	Albumin < 30 g/l
S	Six or more motions per day
T	Tachycardia

K167   C: It is associated with blood group A

Pernicious anaemia is associated with a number of autoimmune conditions and therefore the presence of thyroid autoantibodies does not suggest an alternative diagnosis. Patients with pernicious anaemia are at increased, not decreased, risk of gastric cancer. Antibodies against parietal cells occur in 90% of people with pernicious anaemia but also occur in atrophic gastritis and other conditions, whereas antibodies against intrinsic factor are more specific but only occur in 50% of patients.

Although pernicious anaemia is associated with blood group A this is not necessarily a fact that the examiners would expect you to know. However, they would expect you to reach the correct answer based on exclusion of the other statements.

K168   D: Dermatomyositis

The red papules are known as Gottron's papules and together with muscle pain, muscle weakness and raised creatine kinase point towards a diagnosis of dermatomyositis.

K169   A: Ileocaecal valve

The commonest site of Crohn's disease is in the region of the ileocaecal valve.

K170   B: Ménière's disease

Vertigo, tinnitus and deafness comprise the classic triad of symptoms but patients might also complain of nausea and vomiting.

K171   B: Vitamin C deficiency

This patient has scurvy, a common nutritional finding in poor, elderly and socially disadvantaged groups.

K172   A: Hyperdynamic apex

In chronic aortic regurgitation the increased pre-load and after-load in the left ventricle leads to left ventricular hypertrophy, leading to a hyperdynamic apex.

Due to the reflux of blood from the aorta into the left ventricle, diastolic blood pressure in the aorta is lower than with a normal valve, leading to a wide pulse pressure. The diastolic murmur of aortic regurgitation is best heard with the patient leaning forwards and on maximal expiration. Mitral stenosis causes increasing pulmonary hypertension, which in turn leads to pulmonary regurgitation and an early diastolic murmur that occurs as a result of this is called a Graham Steell murmur.

There are a number of eponymous signs that are associated with aortic regurgitation, some of which should be borne in mind for the exam: Corrigan's sign is a collapsing pulse, de Musset's sign (not Mullet) is head nodding, Quincke's sign is red pulsation in the nail beds, Duroziez's sign is a double murmur heard when auscultating over the femoral pulse. All of these are due to aortic incompetence.

K173   D: Pellagra

The three 'D's of dermatitis, dementia and diarrhoea point towards a diagnosis of pellagra, which is due to nicotinic acid deficiency.

K174   D: Repeated muscle contraction leading to fatigue

In Eaton–Lambert syndrome repeated muscle contraction leads to increased strength. Fatigue on exercise would be more in keeping with a diagnosis of myasthenia gravis. In myasthenia gravis antibodies target acetylcholine receptors at the post-synaptic neurone while in Eaton–Lambert syndrome antibodies target voltage-gated calcium channels.

QUESTIONS ON PAGE 134

K175   B: Hypercholesterolaemia

The metabolic syndrome (also known as syndrome X) is a clustering of metabolic abnormalities which greatly increases the risk of cardiovascular disease and diabetes. There are a number of different classification systems is use, including the WHO and NCEP (National Cholesterol Education Programme) classification systems. The core features include:

– Hypertension

– Central obesity

– Dyslipidaemia (high triglycerides/low HDL)

– Impaired fating glucose

– Microalbuminuria

Patients who have the metabolic syndrome should be fully evaluated and treated to prevent progression of their underlying metabolic abnormalities.

K176   D: Viral upper respiratory tract infections are the most common predisposing factor in the development of the condition

This patient presents with acute sinusitis and exacerbation of pain when leaning forwards is highly suggestive of this diagnosis. The maxillary sinuses are the most commonly affected and CT imaging or MRI is the modality of choice to image chronic sinusitis. The most common organism involved is *Streptococcus pneumoniae* in both adults and children although *Moraxella catarrhalis* is a relatively more common pathogen in children.

K177   B: Eyes deviate away from the lesion

The eyes can deviate towards the side of the lesion, but not away.

K178   B: Worse prognosis if aged over 20 years at presentation

A worse prognosis is associated with patients who present at a younger age.

K179   C: Involvement of the central nervous system is more common in females

The patient is suffering from rheumatic fever, in which an infection with group A β-haemolytic *Streptococcus* leads to an autoimmune inflammatory reaction in susceptible individuals. The modified Jones criteria are used for diagnosing rheumatic fever, which requires two major criteria or one major and two minor criteria to be met in addition to evidence of a recent streptococcal infection.

Major criteria:

- Carditis

- Polyarthritis

- Sydenham's chorea

- Subcutaneous nodules (Aschoff bodies)

- Erythema marginatum

Minor criteria:

- Fever

- Arthralgia

- Prolonged PR interval

- Raised inflammatory markers (ESR/CRP)

- Evidence of group A streptococcal infection

- Previous rheumatic fever

Neurological manifestations of rheumatic fever are more common in females and include Sydenham's chorea, a writhing movement disorder. An ECG might show first-degree heart block (prolongation of the PR interval), which is a minor criterion that can be used for diagnosis. Penicillin antibiotics, salicylates and steroids are all commonly used to treat the condition.

Vesicular breath sounds are the normal breath sounds heard on auscultation and not related to the rheumatic fever.

QUESTION ON PAGE 137

K180   E: Prothrombin time

The prothrombin time is affected by a range of insults on the liver and although it is one of the best measures of hepatic function it is least useful for discriminating between the disease processes leading to cirrhosis.

K181   A: Patients should be screened for past exposure to tuberculosis

Infliximab is an antibody that targets tumour necrosis factor alpha (TNFα), a potent pro-inflammatory cytokine that is central to a number of inflammatory disease processes. Blockade therefore leads to a significant improvement in symptoms and quality of life. It is commonly used within the context of rheumatology but its use is becoming more widespread in dermatology and gastroenterology. Limiting factors in its use include cost and side-effects due to its potent anti-inflammatory properties. There have been a significant number of cases of anaphylaxis associated with its administration and it should therefore be started in a hospital setting. Methotrexate should be co-administered to limit the production of antibodies against infliximab.

K182   D: Bumetanide

Heart failure is often encountered in the hospital and community setting and its management in both the acute and chronic setting should be well known. ACE inhibitors, angiotensin-receptor antagonists, spironolactone, beta-blockers and the combination of nitrates along with hydralazine have all been shown to improve survival in patients with heart failure.

Bumetanide is a loop diuretic and although it is extremely useful in managing the symptoms of fluid overload in heart failure, it has no effect on survival.

K183   E: The bleeding time is usually normal in patients with haemophilia A

Haemophilia A is a disease inherited in an X-linked recessive manner which leads to decreased levels of factor VIII and the father would not be expected to have the disease.

Levels above 5% are associated with mild disease, between 1% and 5% is classified as moderate disease and less than 1% of factor VIII is severe disease. Those severely affected suffer from recurrent spontaneous bleeds into joints and muscles, leading to significant morbidity.

Desmopressin increases the levels of circulating factor VIII and is useful in patients with mild haemophilia but not, in those who are actively bleeding, when prompt administration of recombinant factor VIII is required. Supplementation with recombinant factor VIII is also the mainstay of treatment in patients with haemophilia A.

The bleeding time is a measure of platelet function and is not affected by haemophilia A or B but is affected in patients with von Willebrand's disease, in whom it is characteristically prolonged.

K184   C: Low-molecular-weight heparin

In an intravenous drug user warfarin therapy is fraught with dangers, including non-compliance, interactions and lack of regular monitoring. In such cases daily subcutaneous low-molecular-weight heparin might be preferable as an alternative.

Once-daily low-molecular-weight heparin is also commonly used in oncology patients receiving active chemotherapy as there is concern about multiple potential interactions between chemotherapy and warfarin, making warfarin levels very hard to control and optimise.

QUESTIONS ON PAGE 139

K185   C: Optic neuritis

Inflammation of the optic nerve causes these features. There is a high association between this condition and multiple sclerosis, with optic neuritis being the first presentation of MS in 15% to 25% of cases.

K186   C: Myasthenia gravis

This patient presents with the characteristic features of ptosis and diplopia commonly getting worse as the day progresses, with associated nasal speech. The disease is caused by antibodies against the nicotinic acetylcholine receptor, leading to the characteristic feature of fatiguability. Treatment consists of acetylcholinesterase inhibitors such as pyridostigmine, along with immunosuppressive agents. In severe cases and in myasthenic crises plasmapheresis and intravenous immunoglobulin can be used. In those patients with a co-existent thymoma thymectomy is recommended.

K 187   C: Migraine

This patient is suffering from a vertebrobasiliar migraine, accounting for the neurological symptoms and throbbing headache with photophobia.

K188   B: Systemic lupus erythematosus

Bringing all of the information together, she is most likely to have a multisystem disorder affecting her kidneys (nephrotic syndrome), joints (arthralgia/arthritis) and skin and which also leads to a high ESR but relatively normal CRP.

The most likely diagnosis is SLE, in which the body produces a range of autoantibodies including anti-nuclear antibodies (ANA, positive in more than 95% of patients) and double-stranded DNA antibodies (anti-dsDNA, which are far more specific for SLE).

K189   B: Exchange transfusion

This patient has a sickle chest, which is a haematological emergency. One of the most useful interventions is an exchange transfusion, which removes sickle blood and replaces it with non-sickle cell blood.

K190   A: Bifascicular heart block manifests itself on ECG testing by the presence of right bundle branch block (RBBB) with left axis deviation

Hypothermia leads to bradycardia, atrial fibrillation, PR and QRS prolongation and the characteristic finding is the presence of a J wave, a positive upward deflection after the QRS complex where it meets the ST segment. Delta waves are an indication of pre-excitation and are manifest on the ECG by the presence of a slurred upstroke to the QRS complex.

Complete heart block with a broad-complex (ventricular) escape rhythm is an unstable rhythm and requires placement of a permanent pacemaker. Of the Mobitz heart blocks, Wenckebach (Mobitz type I) is a stable rhythm while Mobitz type II can rapidly progress to complete heart block.

After the His–Purkinje system there are two main branches, the left and right. The left branch divides further into two, the anterior and posterior fascicles, while the right has no main divisions. Bifascicular heart block occurs when the right bundle branch is blocked along with one of the anterior or posterior fascicles of the left bundle. This manifests itself on ECG testing with RBBB and left axis deviation.

In first-degree heart block the delay occurs mostly at the level of the AV node and first-degree heart block with bifascicular heart block is known as trifascicular heart block.

K191   E: NSAIDs

This patient is suffering from acute pericarditis, which is treated with non-steroidal anti-inflammatory drugs. Raised ST segments do not always reflect myocardial infarction and in this case the widespread nature of the ST-segment elevation, along with the patient's young age, should point to pericarditis as the correct diagnosis.

K192   D: Mitral stenosis

Acute mitral regurgitation and not mitral stenosis is a complication of a myocardial infarction, secondary to damage of the papillary muscle.

K193   A: 5

The number needed to treat is an important concept in health economics. In this case 40% of patients died with conventional treatment, whereas 20% died with treatment X and conventional treatment. The absolute risk reduction is therefore 20%.

The number needed to treat to prevent one extra death is therefore $1/20 \times 100 = 5$

K194   C: The screening tool must be highly sophisticated

Screening tools should detect all patients who actually have the disease and a small number of patients who do not have the disease. Therefore they should be sensitive and specific for the disease we are interested in. However, this is an ideal and, in real life, screening tools are far from ideal, with prostate-specific antigen being an example of this.

Although a sophisticated screening tool has a better chance of fulfilling these critieria, it is not vital, with the other features being more important.

K195 A: The patient should have a biventricular pacemaker and implantable cardioverter defibrillator inserted

The patient is 4 weeks post-myocardial infarction and is having runs of non-sustained ventricular tachycardia. He is at high risk of entering into a malignant arrhythmia and should therefore have an implantable cardioverter defibrillator (ICD) inserted as primary prevention. Indications for ICD insertion (available from NICE):

1. Patients with hypertrophic cardiomyopathy and channelopathies such as Brugada syndrome, which carry a high risk of ventricular arrhythmia and death.

2. Primary prophylaxis in post-myocardial infarction patients

   – either with a left ventricular ejection fraction of < 35%, non-sustained VT on a 24-hour tape and inducible VT on electrophysiological tests, or

   – with an ejection fraction of less than 30% with a QRS duration of greater than 120 ms.

3. Secondary prophylaxis in patients who have already survived a sustained ventricular arrhythmia

   – sustained VT or VF causing a cardiac arrest, syncope or if associated with a poorly functioning left ventricle (ejection fraction less than 30%).

However, this patient also has severe heart failure and dysynchrony seen on echocardiography and would therefore benefit from a biventricular pacemaker, which allows cardiac resynchronisation therapy and therefore improves the heart function and decreases symptoms, hospital admissions and mortality compared with optimal medical management. This patient should therefore have a biventricular pacemaker and ICD inserted.

K196 C: 14 units

The maximum recommended alcohol intake is 14 units/week for females and 21 units for males.

K197   B: Physiotherapy

This patient is suffering from an infective exacerbation of COPD and physiotherapy will help in the expectoration of sputum.

K198   E: Tumour lysis syndrome

Treatment of certain tumours, especially those with a high cell burden, causes significant cell death and the subsequent release of intracellular and inflammatory material into the systemic circulation. This leads to the characteristic metabolic complications described in this question, which can result in profound renal failure. It is vital to ensure that at-risk patients are adequately hydrated and have allopurinol prophylaxis.

K199   C: CT scan

The patient is suffering from acute aortic dissection and the imaging modality of choice is a transoesophageal echocardiogram although in reality a CT with contrast is the first-line investigation available to most doctors in the emergency setting.

K200   D: Albumin

Albumin is a negative acute phase reactant (serum concentrations fall in response to inflammation) compared with all of the others, which are positive acute phase reactants (serum concentrations rise).

K201   B: Tennis elbow

Tennis elbow, also known as 'lateral epicondylitis' is a common condition, affecting approximately 8/1000 people. Although classically associated with playing tennis, hence the name, it can occur in a range of occupations and patients. Golfer's elbow affects the medial epicondyle.

K202 A: Autoimmune

This presentation of non-specific symptoms together with a low sodium and high potassium suggests Addison's disease, in which autoimmune destruction of the adrenal glands in the most common aetiology. Patients are classically hypotensive and hypoglycaemic and are often tanned because the increased production of ACTH also leads to increased melanocyte-stimulating hormone (MSH) as both ACTH and MSH share the same precursor molecule.

K203 E: The study is statistically and clinically significant

The study shows that children who watch more than 5 hours of television were found to be at higher risk of having a BMI greater than 30 kg/m². It did not analyse whether there was a dose response, ie if television was watched for longer and longer periods of time during the day would the expected BMI be greater and greater? Due to the nature of children and television it would be impossible to perform the above study in a randomised double-blinded fashion, so option C is false.

The only valid option is E as the data shows a statistically significant result (as seen by the confidence interval) and a BMI of greater than 30 in children is clinically significant (due to their increased health risks). Confidence intervals can be used to denote statistical significance instead of the traditional P value of < 0.05.

K204 C: αFP

Chronic viral hepatitis is a risk factor in developing hepatocellular carcinoma, which is the most likely diagnosis in this patient. The most useful tumour marker is therefore αFP.

Alpha-fetoprotein, together with βhCG, is useful in the diagnosis of certain testicular carcinomas, while CA-125 is useful in ovarian cancers and CA-199 in colorectal and pancreatic cancers.

K205 D: Open angle glaucoma shows a wide racial preponderance, being 5–10 times more common in Afro-Caribbean patients compared with white patients

In the hypermetropic eye the image is in maximal focus in a plane behind the retina while in myopic individuals it falls in front of the retina. Herpes simplex keratitis should be treated with topical aciclovir and not steroids, which would lead to widespread progression of the ulcer, with potentially disastrous consequences. Normal intraocular pressure is between 10 and 20 mmHg and there is a wide racial difference seen in the incidence of glaucoma. Xerophthalmia is a consequence of vitamin A deficiency, which leads to poor night vision and a lack of tear production, leading to keratinisation and ulceration.

K206 D: Physiotherapy should be started early

The patient has developed atelectasis and therefore needs prompt physiotherapy to aid lung expansion and prevent infection.

K207 D: Bronchiectasis

Tram-line and ring shadows are classically associated with bronchiectasis, in which distal airways are permanently dilated due to inflammation or infection. Bronchiectasis is caused by a range of conditions, of which cystic fibrosis is the most well known. Other causes include childhood or severe chest infections, aspiration pneumonia, primary ciliary dyskinesia and allergic bronchopulmonary aspergillosis.

Sarcoidosis classically leads to bilateral hilar lymphadenopathy on chest X-rays, with more severe cases showing interstitial infiltrates and fibrosis. Consolidation leads to air-space shadowing in the region of the lung affected, with visible air bronchograms, which represent air within distal airways surrounded by fluid-filled alveoli.

K208 D: Intrinsic cord lesion

The diagnosis is syringomyelia, in which a cavity forms close to the central canal of the spinal cord. This cavity causes destruction of nerve fibres and accounts for the characteristic symptoms and signs seen in the patient. Of note, coughing or sneezing increases pressures within the cavity, causing it to increase in size, leading to worsening neurological symptoms.

Syringobulbia is a related condition in which the syrinx is present within the medulla of the brainstem, leading to deficits in cranial nerves, dysphasia, pharyngeal and palatal weakness and weakness of the tongue.

A Pancoast tumour is a lung cancer found within the apices of the lungs and it leads to a Horner syndrome on the ipsilateral side due to compression of the sympathetic chain. Apical lung tumours can also invade and infiltrate the brachial plexus, leading to weakness and wasting of the intrinsic muscles of the hands (but this would not be expected to lead to a sensory loss on the trunk).

K209 B: Primary sclerosing cholangitis

The ERCP findings suggest an underlying diagnosis of primary sclerosing cholangitis (PSC). The obstructive jaundice and mass are most likely to be secondary to a cholangiocarcinoma, which patients with PSC are at high risk of developing (in addition to bowel carcinoma).

The vast majority of those with PSC have a previous history of ulcerative colitis, but fewer than 5% of patients with ulcerative colitis are affected by PSC.

K210   A: Lateral medullary syndrome

Lateral medullary syndrome is an examiner's favourite because of its characteristic neurological presentation. It is caused by occlusion of one of the vertebral or posterior inferior cerebellar arteries. It causes ipsilateral cerebellar signs in addition to vertigo, vomiting and dysphagia and a loss of sensation to pain on the ipsilateral side of the face but contralateral side of the body. The lateral medullary syndrome is also known as the Wallenberg syndrome.

Gerstmann syndrome is due to lesions of the dominant parietal lobe in the region of the angular gyrus and leads to four main deficits: left-right disorientation, finger agnosia, dyscalculia and dysgraphia.

K211   D: Cholesteatoma

A cholesteatoma is locally destructive stratified squamous epithelium that can be congenital (with an intact eardrum) or secondary (overgrowth of skin with eardrum perforation). It behaves invasively and can lead to infiltration of the dura, facial nerve (as in this patient) and semicircular canals. Excision is the treatment of choice.

K212   C: Fluid restriction

The patient is suffering from syndrome of inappropriate ADH secretion (SIADH) which is due to either ectopic ADH production or disordered hypothalamic-pituitary function.

The excess ADH causes increased free water absorption by the kidneys and dilutes the plasma, leading to a low osmolality along with lower levels of sodium and potassium in the blood. The urine is conversely more concentrated and has an inappropriately high osmolality, with excessive urinary sodium excretion leading to the biochemical abnormalities seen in the question. Usually a low plasma osmolality would lead to suppression of further ADH secretion, but as this is defective in SIADH a vicious cycle ensues.

Treatment includes fluid restriction, demeclocycline and hypertonic fluid administration with furosemide.

answers

K213   A: Prothrombin complex concentrates

This patient is having a severe gastrointestinal bleed with a significant postural drop and anaemia as a consequence of a grossly elevated INR. In this context vitamin K would not be suitable as it takes 2–6 hours to have an effect, which would be too slow in this patient. Fresh frozen plasma was previously recommended for correction of over-anticoagulation but this has been superseded by the use of prothrombin complex concentrates such as Beriplex and Octaplex. These act immediately but have a short half-life and are therefore taken in conjunction with vitamin K to provide a sustained correction.

Useful guidance on oral anticoagulation and correction of over-anticoagulation is available from the Scottish Intercollegiate Guidelines Network: http://www.sign.ac.uk/guidelines/fulltext/36/section13.html

K214   C: Acute myeloid leukaemia

Auer rods are needle-shaped inclusion bodies found within the cytoplasm of malignant myeloid cells and are almost pathognomonic for acute myeloid leukaemia or pre-leukaemic myelodysplastic syndrome.

K215   D: HSV encephalitis

In this patient the underlying problem is a week-long history of confusion, altered behaviour, headache and pyrexia and, combining these features with the temporal-lobe abnormalities, you should be able to deduce the underlying diagnosis of HSV encephalitis. The ethnicity of the patient should not fool you into thinking that TB is a cause and neither should the history of a cough. There are no features to suggest an immunocompromised state and so JC virus (John Cunningham virus) is not a likely candidate, especially as the clincal picture is not in keeping with its presentation.

K216   E: Initiate warfarin

This question is testing your ability to risk-stratify a patient with atrial fibrillation with regard to his future risk of developing a potentially life-threatening stroke. To do this, a commonly used scoring system is **CHADS2**, which has been validated in patients with atrial fibrillation:

Congestive cardiac failure	1
Hypertension/treated hypertension	1
Age > 75	1
Diabetes mellitus	1
Previous **S**troke or TIA	2

Patients with a score of 0 have a low risk of developing future cerebrovascular disease and no anticoagulation is warranted; patients with a score of 1 are at moderate risk and should be on at least aspirin 75 mg once daily and those with a score of 2 or more are at moderate to high risk and warfarin should be strongly considered provided there are no contraindications. These rules are not concrete and some clinicians elect to start warfarin in patients with a score of 1 if there are additional risk factors or considerations.

In our patient the total score would be 3 (CCF, hypertension and diabetes) and there are no obvious contraindications given in the question so he should be started on warfarin.

QUICK ANSWER REFERENCE

Section 1:
Scenario-based questions

S1.1	E	S9.4	B
S1.2	C	S10.1	A
S2.1	A	S10.2	E
S2.2	E	S10.3	C
S3.1	E	S11.1	D
S3.2	C	S11.2	A
S4.1	B	S11.3	D
S4.2	E	S12.1	E
S5.1	C	S12.2	C
S5.2	C	S12.3	A
S6.1	C	S12.4	B
S6.2	D	S13.1	A
S6.3	C	S13.2	E
S7.1	D	S13.3	A
S7.2	E	S13.4	D
S7.3	D	S14.1	B
S8.1	D	S14.2	B
S8.2	A	S14.3	D
S8.3	B	S15.1	D
S9.1	C	S15.2	C
S9.2	E	S16.1	E
S9.3	B	S16.2	B
		S16.3	D
		S16.4	E

answers

S16.5	A		S24.2	A
S17.1	E		S25.1	D
S17.2	A		S25.2	A
S17.3	D		S25.3	C
S18.1	B		S26.1	D
S18.2	A		S26.2	A
S18.3	D		S26.3	C
S19.1	B		S27.1	A
S19.2	C		S27.2	D
S19.3	A		S27.3	D
S20.1	A		S28.1	C
S20.2	E		S28.2	A
S20.3	C		S28.3	A
S20.4	A		S29.1	E
S21.1	B		S29.2	C
S21.2	D			

S22.1   D

S22.2   D

Section 1:
Knowledge-based questions

S22.3   D

K1	C
K2	C
K3	D
K4	C
K5	B
K6	E
K7	D
K8	D
K9	B

S22.4   B

S22.5   B

S23.1   D

S23.2   D

S23.3   D

S23.4   B

S24.1   C

K10	A		K36	E
K11	E		K37	C
K12	D		K38	B
K13	D		K39	E
K14	C		K40	D
K15	C		K41	D
K16	A		K42	A
K17	E		K43	B
K18	C		K44	C
K19	B		K45	D
K20	D		K46	B
K21	E		K47	E
K22	D		K48	D
K23	E		K49	D
K24	E		K50	C
K25	A		K51	A
K26	A		K52	E
K27	C		K53	A
K28	B		K54	C
K29	C		K55	B
K30	D		K56	C
K31	B		K57	E
K32	E		K58	B
K33	C		K59	D
K34	D		K60	B
K35	B		K61	A

QUESTIONS ON PAGES 58-81

281

K62	A		K88	A
K63	D		K89	B
K64	C		K90	E
K65	B		K91	D
K66	D		K92	C
K67	D		K93	A
K68	D		K94	C
K69	E		K95	A
K70	A		K96	E
K71	D		K97	B
K72	E		K98	C
K73	C		K99	B
K74	B		K100	E
K75	B		K101	C
K76	C		K102	D
K77	C		K103	C
K78	D		K104	E
K79	B		K105	E
K80	A		K106	C
K81	D		K107	A
K82	C		K108	D
K83	A		K109	D
K84	B		K110	D
K85	E		K111	A
K86	A		K112	E
K87	D		K113	A

QUESTIONS ON PAGES 82–106

K114	C
K115	B
K116	D
K117	D
K118	B
K119	A
K120	A
K121	B
K122	C
K123	D
K124	C
K125	B
K126	D
K127	C
K128	B
K129	E
K130	C
K131	B
K132	A
K133	A
K134	E
K135	C
K136	D
K137	E
K138	E
K139	D

K140	A
K141	B
K142	B
K143	D
K144	D
K145	D
K146	C
K147	C
K148	D
K149	C
K150	A
K151	C
K152	C
K153	D
K154	B
K155	C
K156	C
K157	A
K158	B
K159	E
K160	C
K161	D
K162	B
K163	A
K164	A
K165	A

K166	B		K192	D
K167	C		K193	A
K168	D		K194	C
K169	A		K195	A
K170	B		K196	C
K171	B		K197	B
K172	A		K198	E
K173	D		K199	C
K174	D		K200	D
K175	B		K201	B
K176	D		K202	A
K177	B		K203	E
K178	B		K204	C
K179	C		K205	D
K180	E		K206	D
K181	A		K207	D
K182	D		K208	D
K183	E		K209	B
K184	C		K210	A
K185	C		K211	D
K186	C		K212	C
K187	C		K213	A
K188	B		K214	C
K189	B		K215	D
K190	A		K216	E
K191	E			

INDEX

Page numbers preceded by "K" represent knowledge-based questions, those preceded by "S" represent scenario-based questions.

285